ACHIEVEMENT:
Cancer Free for 20 Years

ACHIEVEMENT:
Cancer Free
for **20** Years

Curly Martin

First Published by
Achievement Specialists Ltd

Print ISBN 9870-0-9954858-0-8
Mobi ISBN 9870-0-9954858-1-5
ePub ISBN 9870-0-9954858-2-2

All stories in this book are true but the names of the
individuals concerned may have been changed.

Printed by in the UK by Lightening Source

Disclaimer Notice

This book offers information and guidance only and is not intended as direct advice. I have no control over the way that you use the information contained within these pages – you alone are responsible for the outcomes of any actions that you take, for compliance with local rules and regulations, with medical and governmental obligations and, equally importantly, for all and any of the outcomes of any actions that you take. The author and publisher make no representations or warranties of any kind with respect to this book or its contents. In addition, the author and publisher do not represent or warrant that the information accessible via this book is accurate, complete or current.

This book is my journey; I recommend that you always employ qualified professional specialist advice. Remember, the responsibility for the way that you apply the information contained in this book is entirely yours. The information and statements within this book have not been evaluated and are not intended to diagnose, treat, cure or prevent any condition or disease.

Neither the author nor publisher, nor contributors, or other representatives will be liable for damages arising out of or in connection with the use of this book. This is a comprehensive limitation of liability that applies to all damages of any kind, including (without limitation) compensatory; direct indirect or consequential damages; loss of data, income

Dedicated To Pete

Contents

Acclaim For
Cancer Free For 20 Years

"Whatever your experience of cancer, this book is a route map for survival. It's the story of a busy life suddenly pushed onto a new track at high speed. Full of ideas and good advice, this book is a thoughtful and practical read which sings of endless possibilities: for life is sweet, deserving to be both savoured and fought for."

—ANTONIA SWINSON
Award Winning Business Journalist and Writer,
former Chair Society of Authors in Scotland

"A lovely inspiring, uplifting and funny read. Encourages you to seize the day, every day!"

—PRUE GENT

"A very interesting, amusing, and thought provoking book. A good, easy read. I love the fact that the author did not accredit her health and recovery to any one thing – but all the 'little steps.'"

—JACKIE HAMMANS

"If you have never heard of Curly Martin, you will soon feel that you do know her as your turn these pages. And your knowing will be a joy enough for the price.

In this world there really are takers and givers. Most of us rail against the takers: politicians, power-hungry, inhuman and selfish people who cheat, lie and grasp from us. Fortunately, many of us have collected 'givers' in our circles. Curly is one such and, 23 years on from her own 9 month death-sentence, this latest book from Curly is yet another manifestation of her giving; of herself, of her lessons, learnings, honesty and naked openness to the world. You cannot help but want to turn pages to know more about Curly, her trials, her humor and her positivity in adversity. Most of all, she turns her story into simple tricks of the mind that we can all accomplish easily, improving the quality of our living, and dying.

Curly's book is flush with guidance to have self-mastery in the face of adversity. These tricks of positivity are not just for the fearful and sick, but for all of us; she guides and tempts us to greater psychological wellbeing and well 'being'. She writes, "I think my cancer would have had difficulty growing in a body full of positive energy". Her book is a path to creating wellbeing that should indeed contribute to resisting malignancy or curing, as she did her own.

We all have malignant cells, 'metastases' that occur spontaneously – for most of us, most of the time, these do not lodge and grow into tumours. Thinking well and taking care of our bodies, as Curly suggests, provides all of us with an easily applied set of life-changes that will not only make us feel better every day, but may help save our lives too. The journey is one of both spirit and psychology. As she writes,

"I liberated myself from myself". And the good news is, we can too!"

—PROFESSOR ANGUS MCLEOD, PHD
www.angusmcleod.com

"This book could quite easily make you rethink the way you live your entire life. With the subject matter in hand it is perhaps a tough task to avoid typical cliques, but Curly's writing is inspiring, direct & honest, whilst also being unexpectedly positive from her warm humour and keen wit.

Her story is leagues away from being a 'misery memoir' and instead becomes a celebration of life, with hard earned insights which empower the reader to develop the resilience to tackle serious situations and overcome them to build a better life.

In essence, this book is inspiring reading for anyone involved in any way with a terminal illness, as well a poignant reminder for all of us healthy creatures to fight the temptation to take the richness of life for granted. Highly recommended"

—GRANT WILLCOX
Success & Peak Performance Coach
www.lifesuccesscoaching.net

"Cancer Free for 20 years written by Curly Martin takes you on an a thought provoking journey that gives you hope, inspiration and a different perspective regarding her holistic approach to cancer and her success to being 20 years free of the condition. Curly most certainly writes from the heart and her honesty and topic readability throughout the book is captivating. A must read for anyone that has been affected by cancer either personally or through someone they know.

I feel that the book would inspire hope to someone that has just been diagnosed with cancer. It would offer different perspectives and things to try for the carer of a cancer patient and also that there can be a different outcome regardless of diagnosis. For someone that has just finished chemo/radiotherapy it would provide options/choice and possibly a new focus of things to work towards.

For someone who has been given the all clear it would be interesting, motivating, entertaining and inspiring. For someone that has been told the cancer has returned it can provide hope that even someone with a terminal diagnosis of 8/9 months can still survive and be enjoying life to the full 23 years later.

This book would also be very useful for coaches, NLP practitioners, people working in healthcare, people with other terminal conditions not just cancer as mind-set, psychology and positivity also come into this. Basically anyone would definitely take something away by reading this book."

—KATHRINE SMITH
http://simplypositive.co.uk

Introduction

Since my terminal diagnosis of breast cancer and an aggressive form of lymphatic cancer, over 23 years ago, I am now an international bestselling author, I have become the grandmother of life coach training, I have built a successful coaching business, I am married to a loving husband and we live in a fabulous house in the country. In 1992 I was told I had nine months left to live. This book is the story of my journey. I give you some of the strategies I used to overcome the cancer and how I created an outstanding life. None of this would have happened had I not been diagnosed with cancer. I am not saying this to impress you; I am saying this to impress upon you, that cancer can be the most powerful catalyst of change.

Throughout this book I will be telling you my story at each stage of my journey. What happened, how I handled it, the outcome (if applicable, or if it adds more information for you), what I was offered in the way of medical support, what I did, what extra things happened and any other titbits to inform and amuse you because as you will read here in the book, I believe humour is a great healer.

The book is written with a combination of storytelling and facts mingled together to entertain and educate at the same time. I understand this mingling of fact and fiction is now often known as a portmanteau edutainment. Whatever next? It makes the process sound like some syndrome, not the fun and excitement I like to combine.

If you are in the early stages of your cancer journey, you might find that the many things that happened to me, cause you alarm. Please do not be alarmed; not all the things that happened to me will happen to you. Probably not half of the things will happen to you, especially when you take into account the advances in cancer treatment which have been developed in the interim period. Remember, as you are reading, that I have written this book to reassure you that there can be a future beyond cancer and I hope that I also inspire you to live a full and varied life.

Although the title suggests that my body is cancer free I realise that this statement is strictly scientifically speaking not possible for a living body. What I mean by the title is that I am free of the cancer with which I was diagnosed.

CHAPTER ONE

I DO NOT WANT TO DIE

It is okay to be scared

Help, I am scared and I don't want to die. This is a very natural reaction to the news that you have cancer; I am living proof that death is not an inevitable result when you get a terminal prognosis.

So let me take you on my journey. In the July of 1992, I moved to southern Spain after being made redundant from a very high pressured senior position in a computer manufacturing company. I was really happy to be finally living my dream in Spain, although my boyfriend Pete was not overly happy being left behind in the UK.

Pete came out for a visit in October which did not go well. During the visit he found a very small lump in my right breast. I said very small and I am not joking, most of the time I could not feel it at all. The lump was much smaller than a single petit pois.

I made an appointment with a medical specialist who had been recommended to me, and both Pete and I attended. Looking back, I should have reported this guy to a Medical

Board but at the time I was concerned about the lump and he had come highly recommended – by a man – I need to point out.

We arrived for my appointment and were shown into his surgery. During the consultation he spoke only to Pete, describing me in the third person! He was Egyptian and I was making allowances as I had other things on my mind.

He examined my breasts in front of Pete and then went on to examine my vagina, saying that he was checking to see if there was any spread! I think he must have meant spreading of my legs! After the examination he confirmed, to Pete, that there was nothing wrong with me and that women often make a fuss over nothing. I was so relieved that I did not have cancer that I overlooked the specialist's arrogant and inappropriate behaviour.

In early December I noticed a small lump under my arm. Dr. Faisal Samji, a very dear friend of mine, was coming to stay for a few days so I thought I would ask him about it. When I told him about the visit to the specialist (I say specialist not because I think of him in this manner, only to make it easier for you, to follow the story) I also told him about a further development, an appearance of an underarm lump. He asked if he could examine me. I have to say it is very odd being examined by a close friend. I sat very rigidly, looking at the wall, whilst he had a feel around my breast and armpit. On reflection, I realise I had put him into a very compromising position. In my defence, I did not at the time, consider I would be compromising a friend.

Faisal said that I was not to worry, but that I should go to a different doctor as soon as possible. At the end of his holiday I drove him to the airport and I completely forgot about calling another doctor. I know this seems silly now, but it was coming up to Christmas and Pete and an old girl friend of mine were coming to stay over the festive season. I think it was a combination of him saying 'not to worry' and my not wanting to worry that created this lack of activity. What he meant, I hear you shouting at the top of your voices, is that he was very worried and I should go immediately.

On the 22nd December, after finding that the lumps had increased in size, I remembered that I should make an appointment with another doctor. I went to see an English doctor (who was charming as well as good looking) in San Pedro De Alcántara. He briefly examined me and immediately arranged an appointment with a specialist in a Gibraltar hospital for the following day. Pete had arrived from the UK and my girlfriend had driven from her home in Portugal, so we decided to make the trip to Gibraltar a last minute Christmas shop and off we went. On arriving in Gibraltar they both offered to come with me to the hospital but because I did not consider this visit to be of any significance I told them to go about their shopping and arranged to meet them two hours later outside of the Marks and Spencer shop (yes they do have one in Gibraltar). I had calculated a couple of hours because I thought the hospital visit would only be about 30 minutes and when it was over, I could do my last minute Christmas shopping.

Upon my arrival at the hospital I was examined by a young boy! Well he looked like a young boy! I was 39 years old. After the examination he said that I had malignant growths in my breast and underarm and he wanted to do the operation during the next available surgery slot which was on the 29th December. He also said that I needed chemotherapy treatment and I would have to go to the UK for this as the Gibraltar Hospital did not offer a chemotherapy service. He gave me some contact numbers and in a daze I found myself out on the street completely bemused and befuddled.

I remember confusing the words malignant with benign and thinking I was okay. I had conveniently forgotten the bit about chemotherapy. I now call this form of forgetting, "Hospital Amnesia" which I will be describing to you later in the book. I will also give you some really good tips on how to remember what is said when you are in the hospital. Very useful, I can assure you. Anyway, back to the story. So I was confused between malignant and benign and to be absolutely sure, I went into a newsagents shop and found an English dictionary and looked up the word malignant, which said:

Imminent death!

That was scary and I was terrified.

I felt sick and hot at the same time. The shop walls were closing in on me and I dropped the book and ran out into the road gasping for air. I was frightened and wanted to find Pete, so I rushed around Gibraltar in a panic. Now if you have not visited the island, it is very small, with only one main street, and so you would think it would be easy to find either one of my friends. Well after 30 minutes of searching I was desperate and distraught. I gave up looking for them and I found a little church on one of the side streets and I decided to go in. It was lovely and cool, quiet and reassuring. I just sat there and let the reality of what the doctor had said sink in. I don't remember much about the time in the church except a great sadness and profound hopelessness came over me.

At the appointed time for the reunion, I stood outside Marks and Spencer and waited for them to arrive. Luckily for me, they turned up within a couple of minutes of each other.

'How did you get on?' they both chirruped.

How could I tell them in the middle of a busy Christmas decorated street in a foreign country?

'I have cancer,' I squeaked.

'Oh my God,' said my girlfriend.

'Bloody hell,' said Pete.

'If you don't mind I really would like to go home. That is if you have both finished shopping?'

'Yes, yes we must go back,' they both said.

Now the challenge was that I really did not feel up to driving back to Estepona so Pete drove whilst I tried to answer all their questions. One minute I would be lucid and fine, then the next, I would feel as if I were plunging into an abyss. One minute I was detached and the next, without warning, I would be flooded with emotions and tears would roll down my face.

When I was in the church, I had been thinking about the logistics of having an operation in Gibraltar and the chemotherapy in London, and I knew that I had to speak with my doctor friend, Faisal. As soon as I arrived back home, I called him.

'Hi Faisal, sorry to bother you with this before Christmas, only I have just returned from the Gibraltar Hospital where they told me I have breast and lymphatic cancer and they want to operate on the 29th December.'

There was a deep intake of breath on the other end of the phone.

'And they said that after the operation I would have to come back to London Royal Marsden Hospital for my chemotherapy,' I gabbled.

'If you have to come back for the chemotherapy wouldn't it be better to also have the operation at the Royal Marsden Hospital?' he asked.

'Well yes, I suppose it would but I have not been referred to them.'

'Well, firstly, would you like to have the operation and the chemotherapy in the same place?' he enquired.

'Er.. yes.'

'I can refer you to the Royal Marsden Hospital if you would like that?' he generously offered.

'I would love it, only I don't have anywhere to live, as you know I rented out my flat.'

'You can come and stay with me whilst you sort things out. That's settled then. I will arrange for you to visit the Royal Marsden Hospital and I will call you back with the dates and details,' he asserted.

'Thank you, thank you, thank you,' I stuttered between tears of relief that someone was going to help me.

After I had put the phone down and told them what Faisal had said, we all agreed it was the best course of action to take. Every one of us was unsettled and the evening passed in a haze of disharmony. I cannot remember what we ate only that we all decided to have an early night. I did not want to sleep but agreed with the plan as I wanted some private time to speak with Pete about how it would affect us.

I must mention some more background stuff now, so that you fully understand what happened when Pete and I had our private chat. I had started to have suspicions that Pete was seeing someone else. Let me explain – Pete was a Royal Marine and every year they hold a Christmas Ball where only couples attend. I am not sure if it is one of the many spoken or unspoken rules that only couples are allowed, but singles are not encouraged to attend. I knew the Christmas Ball had taken place because Pete had told me the date of the event before he came to Spain. When I went to pick him up from Malaga Airport (one hour drive), on the journey home I decided I would broach the subject.

'Did you go to the ball?' I asked in a jolly, light hearted, and not bothered about the details, kind of voice.

'Um, well yes,' He said quietly and with reticence.

I now knew he must have taken another woman to the ball.

'What would you like for dinner this evening? I have bought some sword fish as I know you like it. Would you be happy with salad and new potatoes?' I continued in order to stop the conversation about the ball and to let him think that I did not know what was going on. I wanted to consider my next move very carefully, so I played for time.

'Yes that would be great,' he said.

We continued to discuss every boring thing we could think of, to avoid talking about the elephant in the car! That is a way to describe people not talking about big issues.

Now back to the night of the 22nd December. We all went upstairs to bed and once we had closed the door of the bedroom Pete turned to me and said, 'I cannot deal with this.'

I asked him what he meant and he replied, 'I cannot deal with your cancer. I think we should go our separate ways.'

I was stunned. I cannot remember whether I said anything or just turned and left the room. I do remember going downstairs and stoking up the open fire with a couple of logs in preparation for a long night.

I sat on the rug in front of the fire feeling all alone and scared, I just cried and cried. I cried for a solid six hours. You know the type of crying, where you howl, then sob, then gasp for air and it all starts over again. I cried about the injustice of it all, I cried because I did not think I deserved it, I cried because I was only in my thirties. I raged at all the gods. I screamed at the angels for not taking care of me. Quite why they should have taken care of me did not come into this. It was the longest self-pity episode in my history. I hated everyone who was well and healthy. I hated everything in the miserable world.

Then I went on a long and protracted negative rant. I looked and found all the horrible things I had done in my life which had brought this upon me. I dragged up all the lies I could remember that I had told. Each memory brought with it a further outburst of tears. I examined all of my disastrous relationships – there were many! Each failed relationship had deepened my self-loathing. I examined my failure to be a huge success in life. I put under the self-loathing microscope all the work relationships which had failed. Boy was there enough material to fill six hours! I would go round in circles probing all the dark secrets, dismal actions and dreary caves of my miserable little life. I cried and cried and ranted and ranted. In between the sobbing I was stoking the fire with logs and stoking my self-loathing with black memories.

I remember sobbing until there were no more tears. I was fed up with crying and fed up with self pity. At the exact moment of this realisation, the sun was rising and the birds started their dawn chorus. I was so exhausted I just looked at the sun rising and listened to the birdsong. I stopped sobbing and I stopped the hateful negative ranting and I just sat quietly looking and listening. In this exhausted state I turned the first corner.

Sitting there listening to the birdsong and watching the sun rise I started to feel calm and quiet. I was exhausted, so just sitting and being alive was all I could manage. After a while, I cannot say how long because I was not worried about the time of day, it was dawn and that was all I remembered. I asked myself, 'Okay if I die now, how does my life really look? What have I done for the general good of the world?'

Well at first I found I was not able to find anything, so I decided to ask a different question. By the way, this is a brilliant technique to get you from an un-resourceful state into a resourceful state, or even to solve some tricky situations you might find yourself in — ask yourself a different question. I have learnt a lot since 1992 and asking better questions has been a powerful learning on my journey.

Back to the question, 'What have I done for the general good of the world?' As you have probably guessed already, it was a very pompous question and that was the reason I was struggling to find any answers. So I made a very simple change: 'What have I done for the good of somebody else?' Well this was a whole lot easier to answer. I started with very simple small things, like taking a neighbour to the hospital, babysitting a paraplegic girl so her parents could go out for the night, giving a beggar a sandwich, feeding a friend's cat, I am sure you get the idea. I kept on going, I went from friends to neighbours to complete strangers and the list continued to grow. Then I thought about what the people I had helped had achieved or who they might have helped.

This brings to mind what one of my coaches said to me many years later. He trained as a life coach with me and then he went on to create a successful coaching business. I met him one day when I was walking along the beach and he stopped me and said, 'Have you got a minute Curly? I want to tell you something.'

'I always have a minute for you,' I said smiling. He was very handsome, sparkling blue eyes, curly long black hair and a jaunty manner. What girl could resist?

We walked to a bench and sat down facing the beautiful ocean which shimmered on this warm sunny day.

'A while back I had a client who came to me when he was at his lowest point. He had been made redundant and when he arrived home early that same day he had found his girlfriend in bed with his best friend. Well I used all the things you taught me and at the end of our coaching programme he had found a new job, a strategy to find a new girlfriend and he was feeling much better about things. That was about 18 months ago. I often wondered how he was doing.' He paused for breath.

'Well the other night I took my girlfriend out to dinner and in a private room to the side of the restaurant there was a party happening. Half way through the evening a tuxedo dressed man came out of the party. He recognised me and came over and shook my hand. He was the groom and the client I have just told you about. He said he had grown his confidence through working with me and this gave him confidence to start a new relationship. He thanked me and went to get his new wife to introduce me. I was moved by his turnaround and his new found happiness.'

'I am so very proud of you and what a wonderful moment, to know how you have changed that man's life. Well done!' I said, truly touched by his story.

'Well Curly, I did not stop you to tell you how successful I have been; I stopped you to tell you that you will never know how many lives you enrich. You not only change the lives of your trainees and your personal clients, you also change the lives of their clients which you may never have any inkling of,' he said with a big affectionate smile. It was true, I had not considered the ripple effect of the coach training work that I do, until this moment. I tell you this so that you can consider the ripple effects of your kind actions. What do I mean by the ripple effect? When you drop a pebble into a still pond it creates ripples which radiate to the edges of the pond. Thus, if you do a small kind action you may never know how much impact it will create, nor how far reaching it may be.

So back to the story, I kept finding things which cheered me up, to the extent that I said to myself, 'okay, if I go now, I have done some good things.' This simple activity started me on a journey of acceptance which gave me permission to let go. By the time the others had come down for breakfast I had gathered myself together and although still wobbly and weak from no sleep, I was determined not to spoil my last ever Christmas.

SUMMING UP

Looking at this first stage was all about letting go of the emotions in an exaggerated self-indulgent way and then doing some effective reframing.

1   Having a really long and exhausting crying session. Flush it out!

2   Within this session expunging the negative things I had done during my life.

3   Exhaustion point. Becoming tired to the point of no resistance.

4   Asking myself a great question, 'What have I done for the good of somebody else?'

5   Making the list long and detailed so that I convinced myself that I had done some good in my life which led to...

6   Acceptance of current situation.

CHAPTER TWO

LAST WILL AND TESTAMENT

Be prepared, not scared

I am back in London, living with Faisal. What happened before arriving in London I will cover later in the book as there was great learning during this period, only it was not learnt by me until much later in the cancer journey. Prior to my arrival Faisal had arranged the appointment at the Royal Marsden. The appointment confirmed the diagnosis and I was duly booked in for an operation to remove the cancer from my breast and from my underarm.

Operation time

The way I dealt with the operation had a big effect on how quickly I recovered. I am not just talking about the physical aspects of the operation, I am really talking about how I mentally prepared myself and the things I did to keep positive and start the healing process.

Make sure the house is in order

Let's face it, it was hard enough dealing with the fact that I was going into hospital for an operation I knew very little about, with most of the people involved I had not previously met, in an environment I had not been in before. Just the thought made me a bit of a wreck. To overcome the feeling of being out of my depth I decided I needed to distract myself by doing things. I had always found that if I took control back by making myself busy I could calm my nerves. So here is what I did.

Make a list

I made a list of all things I would need whilst I was in hospital including a couple of good easy reading books and magazines. I mention easy reading because before the operation my mind was cluttered with the thoughts of the operation, the other patients in the ward, the nurses and numerous other distractions. After the operation, I thought I might feel rough and not be able to concentrate for long periods, therefore if I had easy reading materials like magazines and short stories, I would not get frustrated by reading the same page in a book many times and still having no idea of the contents.

Even if I was a rocket scientist or Mensa member, the thing I understood was that once I'd had surgery I would feel groggy and my concentration would not be sufficient to read the latest scientific paper on the correct fuel mix for take-off! I thought about listening to audio books which I could buy on tape or CD (nowadays it is much easier with book downloads or streaming a book from your audio book provider). Unfortunately, I did not get around to organising audio books beforehand. The thing is, if I had taken the audio books and a player, the selected books would still have been light and easy listening. I was advised by my nurse that it was normal to lose concentration and was counselled on the need not to get frustrated, as this could slow down my healing and negatively affect my frame of mind.

I prepared and packed all the normal stuff like nightdress, slippers, wash bag, day clothes and make-up bag. Yes ladies, my make-up bag! This was one of the most important of all the casual decisions I made, although I did not realise it at the time. I will tell you more about that later, suffice to say, I am not a daily wearer of make-up. I can go down the street without my lippy on, so it was a weird decision for me to consider, let alone to pack and take my make-up bag with me.

I also needed to sort out with my letting agent (remember my flat was being rented and I was staying with Faisal) how I could get my flat back before the letting contract ended. I realised without knowing for sure, that the possibility of me being able to read, sign and discuss the legal arrangements necessary to enable my flat to be free of tenants in the shortest of time-frames, would be slight or non-existent after the operation. As it transpired this was correct; I could not concentrate on reading a magazine article let alone read and interpret the legal contracts and letters needed to serve notice on my tenants.

Last will and testament

Also as part of the preparation, I had planned to write my will before going into hospital. This part of the story might make you laugh; it always brings a smile to my face. Once I was registered at the hospital and I had unpacked, I realised I had forgotten to get a will made for me. Forgetfulness played a major part in my journey.

I panicked as I really wanted to leave everything in order in the event I did not survive the operation. I asked my nurse if I could pop out but she was not overly happy to let me out of the hospital because she had registered me. I explained that I had not written a will and needed to get a do-it-yourself will kit from the newsagents. The nurse was very understanding and gave me 30 minutes to undertake this task. On reflection, her understanding of my need to write a will could have meant many of her patients had needed one! Thankfully I did not make that connection.

I was really grateful to the nurse for bending the rules and I dashed out to the nearest newsagent, who seemed to have lots of these kits on sale, which was not reassuring. The question, 'should I be worried about the easily accessible will kits?' passed through my mind.

I bought a will kit and returned to the ward within the 30 minutes. I was sitting writing my will when this very handsome surgeon came along with 5 students. He asked me to pop on to the bed and then he noticed the partially written will sitting on the table. He declared 'I had better do a good job as this lady seems to have a very low opinion of my skills!' I was so embarrassed I could not find words to excuse myself. He laughed and saw the funny side of it.

Once he had moved on to the next patient I continued to sheepishly complete my will. The action of completing the will and putting 'my house in order' gave me peace of mind and I felt ready for the future, albeit with trepidation.

Rest and join in

I am not good with general anaesthetics and I was very sick for 24 hours after the operation but the nurses were skilful in keeping my spirits up. The great thing about being sick is that it forced me to rest and this gave my body time to start the healing process. Once I stopped being sick, I realised I was in a ward with some very funny and lovely women. We all chatted and supported each other – it was great to join in the banter when I started to feel strong enough, as this helped with my psychological well-being as well as my physical well-being.

Remember the handsome surgeon? Well, when he came on his rounds, he could not resist saying

'Glad to see you did not need the will!' and all his entourage of students giggled. So did I!

As soon as I was able, I made friends with a couple of the ladies on my ward and I called them my hospital buddies. I was very lucky in that the Royal Marsden Hospital is a cancer specialist hospital and only treats patients with cancer. This meant I was on a ward with people who were all going through the same situation as I was. This removed the need for me to explain what treatment I was in hospital for, giving an added camaraderie amongst all of the patients. We were all on the same journey.

A year later, my best friend was diagnosed with breast and lymphatic cancer and was admitted to a non-specialist hospital without an oncology ward. She woke up from her operation with an oxygen mask over her face and in an isolation ward. This had a profound effect on her and on her recovery. I can only imagine the fright I would have had if I had woken after my operation to find a mask on my face!

I will always make sure that I am booked to be on a cancer specialist ward or cancer specialist hospital if I have any further cancer related operations. I know this decision could affect the rest of my life.

Wash and dress

I realise this sounds a bit odd but the thing I want you to fully understand is that it is easy to slip into the 'I am sick and must stay in bed to show everyone I am sick' pattern of thoughts. The truth is that I can trick my mind into thinking I am healthier than I feel by getting washed and dressed every day. No matter how poorly I felt, and sometimes it would take all day and several attempts, with many rests in-between, I would always have bathed and dressed before evening visiting. I asked my mother to bring in my best silk blouses and pretty skirts so that I would feel well dressed as if I was going somewhere special! And you know what? I *was* somewhere special – getting treatment to heal my special body.

Make-up

It was also very important that I put on my make-up. I needed to make the effort to look good every day. I know it was a bit of a strain some of the days. Looking back I realise it was one of the most important things I did. Every day during my hospital stay, I would manage to put on my make-up. Sometimes I would put my mascara on one eye and then I would need to take a rest. After a short rest I would then apply my mascara to the other eye and then take another rest. Bit by bit I would slowly and purposely apply my make-up to my face before the evening visiting hour. Sometimes this took all day.

Tanning in bed

I had packed a facial bronzer and I used this bronzer every day, so that the face looking back at me in the mirror looked healthy. I looked like I had just returned from a sunny holiday and I would complete the look by doing a full face make-up to include mascara and lippy. The whole process could take hours.

Due to complications, I was in hospital three times longer than expected, so by the time I did leave the hospital I looked like a carrot! It was all about tricking my mind into producing a healthy body to match the visual picture I was showing myself every time I looked into the mirror. It was a great trick and I still use it today if I feel a little under the weather – I find the face tanning cream and slap it on. This works every time for me.

Setbacks

There were many setbacks and how I dealt with them made a big difference to my healthy outcome. I have already told you briefly about the extra 2 weeks I had to spend in hospital which at first really depressed me.

Then one day my friend Lall came to visit me in hospital, having travelled a journey which was completely unfamiliar to her and which included using public transport into and around London, also an unknown for her. She lived in Devon which is over 230 miles from London. When I saw her walking into the ward I was so taken aback it brought tears to my eyes because she cared for me more than her fear of travelling the unknown. This shows great courage as she really did step outside of her comfort zone!

When I mentioned I was feeling low about the setbacks she said: "they are the Universe's way to make you rest so your body can heal itself." It helped me to re-frame my thoughts about setbacks and this in turn helped with the healing. I was not fighting the situation; I was accepting it. Also, her journey was a great inspiration to me – if she could overcome her fear and travel such a long way on her own for the first time, I could overcome my fear of the cancer journey.

Coming out

When I came out of hospital I made sure I rested and that I was kind to myself – this means what it says. I knew I had a burning desire to rush back to "normal life" to prove to myself that having cancer had not affected me. I was invincible. It is great to be thinking positive thoughts but rushing back to work or going shopping the day after coming out of hospital is plain stupid.

I know of people who do just that, come out of hospital after the operation and the very next day go shopping and then they find themselves back in hospital or worse that the cancer has returned. I am not saying this equals that – just, it is sensible to care for your body and this means giving it time and space for rest and relaxation so it can heal itself. I planned to spend the following week after my surgery resting. I decided to rise late in the morning, I had a nap in the afternoon and I went to bed early. I ordered some really funny movies to watch – I explain humour healing and alternative strategies later in the book. I did not fight cancer by using the approach of "being the old busy me equals healthy me." I spent the time being good to me and relaxing, so that my very clever body was using all its energy to heal itself. Either that or I was so poorly I had to rest, the results were the same.

SUMMING UP

Looking at this stage, it was all about being prepared for the operation and for visitors.

1   I wrote a list of all the things I needed to do beforehand, which included what I was going to take to the hospital.

2   I packed some easy reading (could have been easy listening). I remembered to pack some treats as well as all the essential things.

3   As soon as I was able to I made friends with a couple of hospital buddies.

4   I had delivered to the hospital the clothes that made me feel like a million dollars.

5   I got dressed every day in my best clothes.

6   I used facial bronzer and put on my make-up every day.

CHAPTER THREE

WILL MY HAIR FALL OUT?

Chemotherapy creativity

I am still living with friends. It is a little tough as there is nothing like your own home to help with the healing. I was rotating my accommodation to give my generous friends a break from having a lodger. The trouble was, there were times when I just wanted somewhere to howl and it is not as fulfilling to cry silently into a pillow whilst worrying that you might disturb someone. It was a couple of months before I was able to return to my apartment. Lucky for me the letting agent managed to find a lovely flat for my tenants and they were kind enough to move out when they were told the reasons behind my wanting to terminate the letting contract early.

As my cancer was breast cancer which had rapidly spread into my lymphatic system, I was put on to Tamoxifen almost immediately. Tamoxifen is known to block the actions of oestrogen and is used to treat some types of breast cancer. I was taking the drug prior to my operation and I continued with the Tamoxifen for 2 years. On top of the Tamoxifen

I received intravenous chemotherapy (chemo) and it is this form of treatment and my reactions to it that I will share with you later in the book.

Let it roll

When I started my chemo journey I had no idea how it would affect me and I was truly scared. I had already been told my cancer was terminal with a life expectancy of 9 months and I saw no reason to question what treatment was planned for me. The way that I coped with it was to 'let it roll' and what I mean by this, is that I was going to go with whatever was prescribed for me and see what happened. I compare the 'let it roll' with expert boxers, who take the power of a punch by either moving to one side, stepping back or rolling in the same direction of the punch which reduces the impact. They call this 'rolling with the punches.'

My oncology team were clever in the way they would only drip feed me information as and when they felt I needed to know. I guess this process was based on experience and it really worked well with the 'let it roll' approach I was adopting. They did give me some pointers, some of them really horrifying. I was told there was a high probability that I would lose my hair. It was explained to me the different ways this could happen: I was told that my hair could come out in clumps in my hair brush, I could wake up one morning and find most of it on my pillow, or it could just simply fall out a patch at a time.

I was appalled and overwhelmed. The oncology team said that I could have the cold cap treatment, where a cap is fitted over my scalp and then my head would be cooled to freezing point or just below. The cold cap needed to be worn before I had the chemo, during the chemo delivery and after the chemo for a while. I was also told there was no guarantee that I would retain my hair. I was taken to the ward where some of the women were being treated so I could see the process and chat with the other patients. Then I was given time to think about my situation and what I wanted to do.

I had, at that time, long luscious (at least I thought it was luscious) curly hair right down to my shoulder blades and I had worn my hair long for many years. I loved my hair. I was named after my hair (Curly Martin), and what would I be called without it? This was catastrophic; not only did I have this horrible disease, there was a strong possibility I would lose my hair and my identity at the same time. I felt a huge sense of loss and a deep gut churning fear. I knew on a primeval level somewhere in the deep survival recess of my mind that I had to contain this fear or it would overpower me and I would be rendered helpless.

Jack in the box

During one of these fear attacks, a picture of an old wooden box I owned as a teenager came into my mind. It was battered and badly worn and it contained all my teenage confidences. The box had a lock and key and contained my teenage dreams and secrets which, when I put them into the locked box, I felt safe. Thinking about my teenage years brought on another wave of fear and a flooding of tears, which I now call my fear and flood moments. As the wave was flooding over me a thought came into my mind:

'What if I could pop all the negative information about hair on pillows and bald patches on my head into the memory of the box and lock it away for a while, until I could think about it without the fear and flood taking over?'

I did just that! I conjured up the memory of my box. I remember opening the box and looking at some of the things contained therein. A small metal key ring with the letter C, given to me by an old boyfriend, a good luck charm, and my first love letters from a boy called Paul; we kissed at the back of the village hall during a social gathering. I remember that night as if it were yesterday; I was wearing a pair of psychedelic hipster flared trousers and a purple turtle neck shirt which buttoned up at the back! I was a fat (chubby if I want to be kind to myself) teenager and I must have looked outrageous. The thing is; I remember thinking I looked stunning and trendy! I must have, I managed to bag myself the dishy handsome boy called Paul who wanted to kiss me! Anyway, back to the story, I was looking into the box and I imagined that I put a letter with all the hair loss details into the box. Then I closed the lid and locked the box. Doing this small but significant thing helped me keep a hold of my fear and surf over the flood. Every time a fear and flood moment would arrive I would conjure up the box and pop it in!

I know this sounds silly and it is only now, writing this book, I feel able to share this with you. I realise now that the silly things I thought about and I did in the secrecy of my mind or home, along with all the other weird and wonderful antics I ventured into, when added together, played a big part in my dealing with and healing of cancer. I did many silly things, which under normal circumstances I would be too embarrassed to tell you.

I call it Jack in the Box because every time some negative thought popped into my head I would use my imagination to shove it back into the box – sometimes I even imagined sitting on the box to keep it in there!

Another idea, supplied by one of my trained coaches, Grant Willcox, is to think of a negative thought shredder and put the idea, negative thoughts, negative feelings etc., into the shredder. I think this is a great idea and I will give it a go the next time I want to get rid of negative thoughts or feelings.

Try it on for size

The hospital told me that I would be sent a wig in the post from some central NHS department. I did not want to wait until the NHS wig came or my hair had fallen out, so I took the initiative (again taking some control which I think helped the healing). I made appointments with wig shops and talked to a wig maker. I took a fun friend with me to the shop and we giggled as we tried on different wigs. Doing this enabled me to share my fear and turn it into fun.

The assistants in the wig shops were very kind and joined in the fun. Eventually I bought a wig in a style I would never normally be associated with, a blond bob! We all agreed the wig really suited me and I felt I was ready for the hair loss. I was so very glad I had visited the wig shop as the NHS wig the hospital sent was dull, middle aged and looked ghastly on me. Had the NHS wig been my first contact with wigs, I would have been very upset and this in turn would have negatively affected my healing process.

Put a hat on it

I have a friend called Prue who is really good with scarves and she came along one day and we played with scarves until I was confident I could tie a couple of differing styles of scarf over my head. I also spent one afternoon looking at various different types of head gear, hats, beanies, bobble etc. This meant I was prepared and not waiting for the effects of chemo before doing my research. There are lots of videos on the internet of how to tie head scarves which I have since watched and played around with.

Hospital amnesia

Prior to going into the hospital in the early days of my cancer journey, I thought about what important questions I wanted to ask the oncologists. As soon as I passed over the threshold of the hospital I would lose all sense of self and although to an outsider I would appear to be lucid and competent, actually I was not. I would ask a couple of questions and look as if I was listening to the answers but the truth of the matter was I would not be able to retain the information. I do not know why this happened, it just did. I could not remember what I really wanted to ask, nor would I retain the things the medical staff told me.

I called this experience Hospital Amnesia because that was what happened. Outside the hospital I would be a normal human being (relatively speaking – actually if my relatives were speaking about me they probably would not put my name and normal in the same sentence) but once inside the hospital I became mentally dependant and compliant. This was a major setback and an enormous irritant to my mother. She came to live with me and support me for a short while, once I had moved back into my apartment. She would come with me to the hospital and wait for me in the waiting room. When she asked me what was said, or what were the answers to the questions we had talked about, I could not remember. I could not remember all the questions I wanted to ask nor could I remember the answers to the questions I did manage to ask!

I instinctively knew it was important to feel I had some control and with this in mind I used to prepare for the each chemo meeting with the oncology team. I mentioned that I had called this reaction hospital amnesia, and I have heard since from medical professionals that forgetfulness is fairly common.

To overcome this handicap I would write down all my questions on a large A4 size pad of paper, leaving a couple of line spaces in-between questions and a few lines at the end for things the oncology team told me. When I arrived for my appointments I would tell the oncologist that I had a list of questions and I needed to write the answers down along with whatever they needed to tell me. The oncologist was always happy for this to happen even though it took longer for the sessions. Actually, in the long run it probably saved time because I was not asking the same questions time and time again.

The freedom to ask questions changed the chemo combination I was given. After each intravenous chemo and in-between, I would feel really nauseous. When I mentioned this to the oncologist I was told I was on anti-sickness tablets and it should settle down. Well, this did not happen and I had a very strong intuition that it was the sickness drugs which were making me feel sick! The next time I visited the hospital (with my list) I asked the oncology nurse, 'What would happen if I stopped taking the anti-sickness pills?'

The nurse said, 'You will feel very sick.'

'Will that affect the efficacy of the chemo?' I enquired.

'No, it will not affect the impact of the chemo, it will only make you feel very nauseous,' she said.

'Well I feel sick anyway so can I stop taking them and see how I get on?' I implored.

'Yes you can, and if you feel sick you can start taking them again,' she replied.

From that day onwards, I did not take another anti-sickness pill. As soon as I stopped taking the tablets, the nausea stopped and I felt a hundred percent better. I was exhausted by the chemo but I did not also feel nauseous and I was not physically sick. Result!

Rest to recuperate

Chemotherapy is cumulative, which means as you receive each dose it builds on the previous doses. This meant at the beginning I felt okay after the first session and was wondering what all the fuss was about. Towards the middle and end of my programme I would find that for two or more days after the treatment I would feel more than tired, sort of limp and lifeless, heavy and a bit depressed. This is natural and I found that I could deal with this by accepting it and planning to spend the days after the chemo quietly.

I would plan to rise late in the morning, have a nap in the afternoon and go to bed early. I did not fight it by being the old "busy me equals healthy me." I spent the time being good to myself and relaxing so that my very clever body was using the energy to heal itself rather than using the energy for walking about. I planned lazy healing days and put them in my diary beforehand so I was reminded to say 'no' to any requests to go partying on those days.

Being selfish

I was born under the astrological sign of Libra. Whether you believe in this or not, there are two traits which are said to be strong within people born within the Libra dates. One is not being able to make a decision (it has taken me 23 years to finally decide to write this book!) and the other is the desire to please people and make friends with everyone. Therefore being selfish, and by this I mean putting self-interests before other people's wants, did not come naturally to me. However, when it is a matter of life or strong possibility of death, it was a no brainer.

I had to learn very quickly how to be selfish and I learnt that this was incredibly important. During the treatment my immune system was seriously compromised, which meant that my immunity was very low and I was not able to deal with viruses and bacteria. The oncologist had warned me that this would happen and that I was to avoid contact with people who were carrying, or who had been in contact with someone who was carrying, a virus or bacterial infection.

I learnt the habit of washing my hands and face immediately when I returned from an outing, to reduce the risk of infection. Even today, I use a viral and bacterial hand sanitizer because I have become used to reducing risk. It has meant that I do not seem to have many colds or flu and if occasionally, as has happened, I catch an infection, it will usually last for a reduced number of days and is less potent. What a great positive learning to come from the difficult cancer journey.

During the chemo time, I would insist that anyone who visited me wash their hands on entering my apartment and that they do not visit if they had any signs of illness. To be fair, everybody was brilliant and even though there were times we had to cancel at the last minute either because I was not well or they would have an infection, nobody took offense.

In the chapter about radiotherapy I will tell you about when I nearly died because I had let my guard down. This was a salient learning for me.

No cap

Going back to hair loss, I thought I would just finish with my choices. I did not fancy the cap treatment as some of the women said it was a bit hard going and as there was no guarantee of success, I declined the cap treatment. Prior to cancer I held senior positions in global companies and part of my role would involve visits to customer sites. With a name Curly Martin, when I arrived at some of my clients' business sites I would be greeted with, 'Well, well, well. I thought you would be a short bald bloke not a woman!' With this in mind I joked with myself that if I lost my hair, the old clients would be right. Well at least right about the bald head!

As soon as I was told about the hair loss, I booked an appointment with a hairdresser and had my long curly hair cut into a very short spikey style. I did not wash my hair with shampoo for the duration of the treatment and to keep it clean I would simply let the shower water run through it. To dry my hair I just gently patted my head with a towel and let it dry naturally. I was one of the lucky ones, as I did not lose my hair, although it did thin out quite a lot and even that was alarming. My heart and love goes out to all the women and men who lose their hair.

People deal with cancer treatment in many different ways. As you know I was diagnosed way back in 1992 and the treatments were quite harsh in those days. As the chemo programme progressed so the effects on my body escalated. Nowadays, there are very effective treatments which sometimes mean that no radiotherapy or chemotherapy is needed to eradicate the cancer. Many more people are surviving this disease which is great news for all concerned.

SUMMING UP

Chemotherapy can have profound effects on the body.

1   Putting negative thoughts into an imaginary box helped me keep a control of my fear. I called it a Jack in the Box.

2   Another idea on how to deal with negative beliefs is to create a mental negative thought shredder.

3   I rested to recuperate as I knew it would speed up my healing process.

4   Wigs and hats can be fun; I made a day out of the search for one.

5   Being selfish is an *absolute* must when it comes to infections.

NB: I only took Tamoxifen for 2 years as you already know, but I heard about this research and wanted to share it with you as it gives hope.

Professor Jack Cuzick, of Queen Mary University London, conducted a study using 7,000 women and his results revealed women taking Tamoxifen for 5 years had a 30% reduction in risk with a protective effect lasting up to 20 years.

CHAPTER FOUR

RADIATION KILLS

The radiation ride

I am truly hoping the topic of this chapter will soon be void because since my treatment, the years of research and development have made huge improvements in delivering radiotherapy. The latest enhancement being one single dose of radiotherapy delivered by new equipment called the probe. As I am writing this chapter, the probe is currently being used on some breast cancer patients. I will write more about this near the end of the chapter. So what happens first?

Tattoos

Yes, there is a strong chance you will be tattooed! I was really surprised when the oncology nurse told me I would be having a tattoo. I had been tempted to have tattoos when I was a teenager, only my parents thought nice girls did not have them so wanting to be a nice girl, I did not have one.

The reason why you have to undergo a tattoo is because the radiographer needs to be able to line up the radiography equipment in the exact same place every time you have the treatment. The radiographer and nurse work together to line up the machine and once they are absolutely sure of the measurements, you are given tattoos, ensuring that you receive the radiotherapy exactly where you need it. It is called targeted radiotherapy. Radiotherapy permanently damages the DNA of cancer cells, and the healthy tissues around the cancer can also undergo temporary cell damage from the radiation. Notice the use of the words, "temporary cell damage", this is because these cells are normally able to repair any DNA damage and return to growing normally. The use of tattoos contains the area affected.

I was horrified with the thought of being tattooed and I had some sleepless nights because of it. However, when I saw the tattoos, they were very small little dots (pin pricks) and look ironically a bit like a tiny skin mole only blue/black. Having the injections for the tattoo did not hurt; in fact I cannot remember it at all. The thing is that the precision radiotherapy could only take place with the markings and when I fully understood the reasons behind the tattoos it was easier to accept.

If I'd already had tattoos, I might have considered designing a new one to incorporate the radiotherapy markings as a commemorative gesture. I would have had to wait until I had completed my treatment and my skin had properly healed, checking with my doctor before taking this action. Once I had finished the radiotherapy a new tattoo could have been a celebration of getting through to the end.

At first, I did not like the reminder of the effects of the radiotherapy and if I was not such a wuss (coward, wimp),

I might have considered having the tattoos removed. But the thought of their removal filled me with dread and it was especially daunting to consider having treatment which was completely unnecessary, as the tattoos were not visible when wearing normal clothing.

Now I am happy with my tattoos. They remind me of the challenges of my life, the great changes that the cancer brought and they are a true celebration of my success.

As the radiotherapy came after the chemotherapy, I had more confidence about asking about things I did not know and I also was confident in taking in my list of questions. As before, during the chemotherapy, I wrote down the answers and any further information the radiographer offered. I always found what worked well for me was being fully prepared beforehand and taking the time to write down and then ask questions to find out as much as possible about how each stage could affect me. The radiologist and nurses will always add the caveat that everyone responds differently, and this is true. It is just that I am curious and have a yearning for learning, especially when it is about my body.

One of the things I was told, yet I did not fully take it on board at the time, was that the radiotherapy process was going to get progressively harder on me in two separate ways: the first is utter tiredness and the second effect was a psychological one.

Hitting the wall

Unlike when I had chemotherapy where the tiredness grew slowly with the treatment, with radiotherapy, I found I was going along like a puppy, when without any warning I would hit a wall of tiredness and immediately have to stop and rest. When I say immediately, I do not use the word idly, I found I would be doing something, washing the dishes, putting clothes away, any job, and all of a sudden, bam! To call it tiredness does not do the feeling justice, neither would selecting the overused word, exhausted (used by women who have spent the day shopping!) encapsulate the overall experience. I suppose deadbeat or wiped out are better descriptions of the experience. I think on reflection it was the suddenness (not expected) and the force of the debilitation which I remember the most.

It is obvious there would be physiological changes to my cells during the radiotherapy and because I had several treatments, the effects would be cumulative; there was a big chance that I would develop some skin blisters and peeling. Although I was told at the start of the treatment that there might be some skin blistering, I really did not take this information on board. During the whole cancer journey I had a clever little knack of deleting, or not storing, the horrible information; I think this was a coping mechanism.

I cannot remember if I was told radiotherapy would be like being out in the African midday sun without clothes, shade or sun screen, or whether I had blanked out the information. I would have been more geared up if I had asked to see some pictures of the progression. I know what I have just said is contradictory but, because I had no idea (for whatever reason – me blocking or not being told) I did not take as much care with my skin as I should have.

I have no way of knowing, if I had used more skin cream or skin care regimes, I would not have blistered so badly, it's just, if there were some pictures of cared for skin and skin left to its own devices I might have taken more notice. Anyway, towards the end of the radiotherapy my skin blistered and the blisters split, spewing out smelly pus. This was not pleasant and the good thing about it was that it was temporary and there was no scarring.

The second effect is psychological

I really was not prepared for the dips in my emotional state during the radiotherapy. I am not sure if it is because the radiotherapy came at the end of my treatment and I was already pretty psychologically exhausted, or if it was as a direct result of the radiotherapy. I would just burst into tears for little or no reason. It would happen anywhere, I would just feel so low and helpless and the tears would roll down my cheeks. The crying was not the howling I did at the beginning when I was first diagnosed. That type of crying has energy and vibrancy. No, the tears were silent and powerless, just like the way I felt. I do not remember having negative depressing thoughts; I just remember the tears rolling down my cheeks.

How I dealt with the dips

If I was at home when one of these tear dips washed over me I would watch a funny movie. At the start of the movie, I would not find it funny but gradually, as I was becoming distracted from my self-pity, I would start to smile and before the end of the movie I would start to laugh. If I was going out of the house I carried a recording of something that I found funny which I could play on the go. At that time I did not know about the power of laughter to heal the body by boosting my immune system and I will tell you more about that in a later chapter.

Being careful

This is incredibly important. During my radiotherapy treatment my immune system was compromised, very low and not able to deal with viruses and bacteria as it does normally. This was especially true because I had already been through chemotherapy.

I was extra vigilant when shopping, as I did not know who had touched the products before me. Here is a stomach churning example of the need to take great care. One day I was washing my hands in the ladies' toilets when an elegantly dressed woman came out of one of the cubicles where she had defecated. She opened her handbag, took out her lipstick and applied it to her lips, and then she brushed her hair before promptly walking out. She had no intention of washing her hands. I followed her out, putting a paper towel over my hands so that I could open the door. I am sure some of my readers will smile at this, having done something similar, opening toilet doors without making skin contact.

This disgusting woman went straight to the fruit counter and proceeded to squeeze the fruit to see if it was ripe! Well you could have knocked me down with a feather. I was horrified. Let me be clear here, this is not an isolated case; this was the first time I had consciously observed other toilet users. After years of observation, I am sadly aware that for every hand washer, there is a non-hand-washer.

There have been times in the past when I would buy an apple and eat it without washing it, and I have often popped a raspberry or strawberry into my mouth without first rinsing it under the tap. From that day, no matter what, I have washed or peeled fruit before consuming it.

Back to the point it is important to be vigilant about containing the spread of bacteria and viruses. I was pretty good with this, but towards the end of my treatments (when I was at my lowest resistance) I was caught off guard. An Argentinian friend of mine had just returned from a long visit to her home country with her children. I had spoken to her on the phone before visiting and asked her if everyone was healthy, to which she replied that they were. We had a lovely lunch and during the dessert she casually mentioned that her two children had contracted mumps whilst they were in Argentina. I was a little alarmed, but she assured me all was fine. I went home and promptly forgot all about it.

One morning, a couple of weeks or so after my visit, I woke to find I had difficulty breathing and my face and neck were swollen. I rang Faisal's surgery (Bush Doctors) and left a message for him to call me after seeing his morning patients.

The phone by my bed rang, it was Faisal. 'Hi Curls,' he chirped.

'Sorry to bother you, only my face and neck are swollen and I am having difficulty taking deep breaths,' I puffed.

'Are you still having radiotherapy?' he enquired.

'Yes I am, but I think it could be mumps as Carmella's kids had mumps when they were in Argentina,' I managed.

'Can you drive to my place?' he asked.

'Yes I think so. Do you think it could be mumps?' I puffed.

'Good! Let yourself in and go straight to bed. I will be back as soon as I can,' he instructed.

I got out of bed, dressed and drove to his home, which was in Shepherds Bush, hence the name of his surgery – Bush Doctors.

As the day wore on, my breathing became more and more laboured. Eventually, I heard two voices coming up the stairs. Faisal entered the room. 'How are you?' he enquired.

I went to speak but I could not get a word out. Faisal looked concerned and said, 'I have brought one of my partners with me as I wanted a second opinion. Is that ok? Can I call him in?'

I nodded.

He came in, did a quick check and both of them left the room.

Faisal came back into the room. 'Get out of bed, and put a coat on over your night dress, as I am taking you straight to the Royal Marsden. I have called them and they are expecting us,' he said.

Looking back I think I should have been panicked but I was too poorly for that and was happy Faisal had taken control of the situation.

When we arrived at the hospital there was quite a commotion with comings and goings of doctors and lots of listening to my chest. The reason for all the concern, I learned later, was due to possible lung collapse or damage from the radiotherapy. It turned out I had mumps! The moral of the story is that I should never let my guard down and I should always err on the cautious side. I ought not to have visited my friend at a time when my immune system was so low, regardless of the situation.

We have come to the end of the radiotherapy chapter and I just wanted to mention the huge advances that have taken place in delivering radiotherapy. There is a single dose radiotherapy treatment for breast cancer patients using new equipment called the probe. The radiotherapy is delivered immediately after the removal of the cancer; during the operation, before the wound is closed. This approach is proving to be very successful and I can see this idea being developed across the board of all types of cancers over the next few years. How wonderful to replace the long protracted treatment plan I had to go through, replacing months of radiotherapy with a single dose during the operation. Yippee!

SUMMING UP

Radiotherapy is changing for the better and the advances will change the treatment process dramatically over the coming years.

1   I learnt as much as I could so that I was fully prepared.

2   Blistering occurred from the radiotherapy.

3   It soon healed.

4   I did not take good care of my immune system and it was compromised.

Nowadays I always use a viral and bacterial hand sanitizer on my hands and face before leaving the house, whilst out and about and immediately upon return. If I was sick again I would insist that anyone who visits me uses a viral hand sanitizer and I would request that they do not visit if they have any signs of illness.

CHAPTER FIVE

SETBACKS

The stumbling blocks on the road to recovery

Sadly there will be setbacks in your recovery and if you view them as only small stumbling blocks on the road to recovery, it will help. For me, each individual setback seemed far worse than a stumbling block at the time.

I am not going to go through all the setbacks because it would be boring and unnecessary to the telling of my tale. I will tell you about the ones that had a lasting impact. There will be setbacks for almost everyone who is experiencing cancer and the setbacks will be as different as the people experiencing them.

Tea trolley

The first setback came immediately after the operation, only I did not realise it was a setback nor that it was unusual at the time. Remember, I told you I was pretty sick with the anaesthetic and it took me a couple of days before I was interacting with the other people on the ward. Well that was not the only little challenge I encountered. Because the cancer had metastasised (lots of new words for me to learn, this one means that the cancer had spread to other parts of my body) into my lymph nodes (little clearing houses for the lymphatic system) this meant I had to have the lymph nodes removed from my underarm, leaving only three nodes behind. There are approximately twenty lymph nodes under each arm and this means that I had seventeen removed.

For some reason, the area where the incision was made did not want to heal and this extended my stay in the hospital. The great thing about this was that I had no idea how long a normal stay after the operation should take, so I was not perturbed by the length of stay, and anyway, I did not have my own home to go to at that time. My thoughts were along the lines that the longer I was in the hospital the better because it reduced the time spent inconveniencing my friends.

In the end I was so used to the routines on the Ellis Ward that I would offer to take the tea trolley around to break up the monotony of the day and it gave me extra opportunities to chat with the other women in this female only ward. Don't get me started talking about the importance of single sex wards as I am unlikely to stop.

Leaking armpit

Eventually, I was released only to run into the next setback, a leaking armpit. The lymph was building up and burst out through the hole where the saline drip had been. I had to go back into the hospital. I had a couple of extra sleepovers in the hospital until it was all sorted. The stays in hospital reduced the burden I was putting on my friends as a guest who outstays her welcome. I believe it was Benjamin Franklin who famously said "Guests, like fish, begin to smell after three days." I did not want to start to smell, which leads me nicely onto my next setback.

Constipation

I cannot remember if I was told I could develop constipation or not. I had been prescribed a codeine based pain killer and in those days I was not a vegetarian, nor did I know about keeping one's body hydrated.

I had gone to Devon (I am a Devonian) to stay with my mother for a few days during my chemotherapy and I started to feel unwell. Okay, I was not feeling great anyway but what I mean is that I felt a lot worse than the normal unpleasant feelings associated with the treatment. Prior to the cancer I had been prone to irritable bowel syndrome and I thought I was going through one of these attacks. Only the pain got worse as the day wore on and I kept trying to be sick but could not produce anything other than bile. I ended up on my hands and knees as this was the only comfortable position I could find. I moaned in pain. Mother called her doctor. When he arrived he assessed the situation, taking into account the cancer treatment and called for an ambulance.

Mother lives in the middle of Devon in a small hamlet, down narrow lanes and so the Air Ambulance was scrambled. The helicopter landed in the adjacent field and I was duly fitted onto a stretcher which was slid through a tunnel at the side or back of the helicopter. I went in head first so that my head was sticking out in the cockpit with the two paramedics. My body was encapsulated in the tunnel. I remember one of the paramedics chatting to me, pointing out landmarks (not that I could see them, I was looking at the ceiling of the helicopter) as we flew to Derriford Hospital in Plymouth. After many examinations, it was determined that I had chronic constipation, known as faecal impaction. They did not see this as a big problem and sent me home the following day.

As it happens, I had an appointment at the Royal Marsden that same week so I travelled back to London and attended the clinic. I was still in considerable pain and my bowels had not performed. Luckily for me the hospital admitted me to the Ellis Ward and four days later, after several enemas and two or three combinations of enema with some oral medicine, I finally was able to relieve myself. Apparently, constipation can kill you and this may have been the reason the Royal Marsden took the situation seriously. It is a long standing joke in our family that the only family member to travel by Air Ambulance had constipation. Don't you just love families?

Lymphedema

Lymphedema, in layman's terms, is localised fluid retention and tissue swelling. In my case, this was as a direct result of the removal of my underarm lymph nodes. When the little clearing stations (lymph nodes) are removed from the underarm the lymph just seems to puddle. The fluid has to go somewhere so it collects in the arm and underarm area which as a result becomes swollen. The oncology team did say this would happen but I was not prepared for the pain and the cumbersomeness of it. I am not going into the medical or physical explanations or descriptions of lymphedema; I am going to explain what my experience of this was and how I managed to overcome the problems and how, to this day, I am keeping the boogie lymphedema at bay.

The nurses told me to take very great care with my hand and arm as any infection, no matter how small, would cause a swelling. One day, I cannot remember exactly what happened, my right hand and arm ballooned and became very painful. I could have cut myself, I may have been bitten by an insect or it could have been a result of very hot weather. I went to the Royal Marsden Hospital and I was sent to their lymphedema clinic. Once there the nurses measured my arm and issued me with this very ugly brown elastic support sleeve and a separate brown support fingerless glove. I cannot stress how ugly and uncomfortable these supports were. I tried everything I could think of to reduce the swelling to avoid having to wear these supports.

Briefly, to aid your understanding, the lymphatic system consists of lymphatic vessels that allow movement of a clear fluid called lymph to travel towards the heart. There are two functions of the lymph system: one is to help the blood veins by moving fluid (in the form of lymph) back to the heart and the other purpose is that it contains lymphocytes (white blood cells) which are necessary for a healthy immune system, as it removes cell waste, protein and bacteria. The lymph nodes act like a recycling filtering plant, where waste goes in, gets filtered and is moved on to different destinations. The key to understanding the lymphatic system is that it has no pump, so it only moves around the body when the body is moving.

I seem to remember the nurse saying that it helps to elevate the limb. Misquoting from a poem by Alexander Pope "A little knowledge is a dangerous thing." Well, with this in mind, I thought I could help the drainage of the lymph by holding my arm up, which was not only uncomfortable but as soon as I lowered it the lymph would drop back down. I had a lot of pain and discomfort at night so I found an old sling and nailed it to the back of the bed headboard much to Pete's chagrin (I will explain how Pete came back into my life in chapter 8). That night I thought I had found the answer to the world's lymphatic drainage problem and thoughts of possible Patent Office registration and loads of money flooding in, kept my spirits high. Settling into bed lying on my back, I raised my right arm behind my head and put my hand into the sling in the direction, from headboard towards the foot of the bed. This action was to reduce my hand slipping out of the sling because it was pushed against the headboard thus offering me a bliss filled sleep that was undoubtedly coming my way.

Twenty minutes later, whilst Pete was gently snoring, I realised I could not get comfortable. My hand had gone numb and it felt cold. Although I could not see it in the dark, I instinctively knew it was turning blue through loss of blood. The Heath Robinson lymphatic drainage sling (William Heath Robinson was an Englishman who is known for his drawings of outrageously complicated mechanisms for achieving simple tasks, which is what I seemed to have created) was having some technical hitches (hitch being the word of the moment, as I was hitched up to the bed) but because I had put my hand in the sling from back to front I could not get it out. I was unable to use my left hand to free it because it would not reach due to the positioning of the sling. After several attempts to extricate myself from my fabulous world saving device, I had to shout for help before my hand dropped off. So it was back to the drawing board for me.

The thing is the nurses told me that I should be careful with my arm and hand and not to do anything strenuous, nor do gardening etc. without gloves, as a cut or splinter would activate the lymphatic system and swelling would occur. At first, when I had the swelling I started to call my right arm, 'my bad arm'. I soon realised that the arm was not bad itself, and if I kept calling it by this name, I would begin to dislike the arm which would not help with the healing process. So I renamed it my "special arm" and that seemed to work, as I no longer resented it but considered the extra needs of it. You can guess where this paragraph is going! Yes, I did not have the ugly brown elastic glove on my hand when I went to open our wooden gates at the side of the house, hey presto, splinter and swelling of my special arm.

Manual lymph drainage

My best friend Annie told me about her friend, a nurse called Anne Williams, who was studying a new form of lymphatic drainage. Anne Williams had travelled to Germany to study the Manual Lymph Drainage (MLD) techniques which were pioneered by two Danish doctors, Drs. Emil and Estrid Vodder, known as the Vodder Technique. She needed practice patients to qualify and my friend asked if I would be interested. Well quite frankly I would have swung off the chandeliers if I thought it would ease the pain and discomfort. Actually, I did swing from the sling, now that I am thinking of it.

I jumped at the chance and as soon as was possible I arranged to have this new form of massage. It worked like a dream. Within a couple of sessions my right arm and hand were reducing in size and the pain was easing. After I had completed the whole programme with Anne Williams, my arm was nearly back to normal and the pain had gone. I was ecstatic. Anne then taught me how to perform this massage on myself, so that if at any time she was not around, I could administer the MLD on myself.

I was, and still am, so impressed with the results of MLD that I decided to fit the massage into my daily showering routine. MLD is a feather-light gentle massage and the water of the shower produces a gliding effect when I run my left hand over my special arm. I still do this today. I have had many occasions to use the MLD on myself, as being in a very hot climate, or a sunny day in England (a rare and wonderful treat) always causes my special arm to swell. If this happens I simply turn on a cold shower, stand under it to reduce my core body temperature and perform the MLD which always manages to reduce the swelling. I am such a lucky woman and I am eternally grateful to Anne Williams, who is now Dr Anne Williams and very well deserved. You can read all about her here: *http://www.mldtraining.com/*

Weight gain

I have always been a little over weight. When I was a teenager, a boy I fancied used to call me "jelly arse" which, because I had a personality to match the size of said appendage, did not offend me. It was only in my late teens that I became body conscious and my weight yo-yoed as I tried diet after diet with a variety of degrees of success. One day, when I was berating the fact that I had cancer, a friend said that I should look on the bright side, as having cancer would most certainly mean that I would lose weight.

'Oh will I?' I asked interestedly.

'Yes, most people do,' my friend replied.

Well, I thought the saying that every cloud has a silver lining will be true if I can lose weight during this ordeal.

Two stone later, I turned out to be the exception that proved the rule, whatever that means. I simply piled on the pounds. So instead of losing weight, I gained it.

Sickness

When I had the chemotherapy cocktail there was also within the cocktail an anti-sickness drug. I took this drug as instructed but instead of relieving the feelings of nausea I constantly felt sick and this was seriously reducing my appetite. I asked if it was essential that I take the tablets and the nurse emphasised that they prevented nausea. I explained it was not working for me and she agreed I could stop taking them. Almost immediately I no longer felt sick.

And because I had worked out that the anti-sickness pills caused the nausea which was preventing me from eating, once I no longer had to take the tablets, I could tuck in happily and heartily to all foods, which is what I did. It has taken me years to get the excess weight off but I do not mind as I am alive and able to work on it. I would rather be fat and alive than skinny and dead. Can you be skinny and dead, or should that be dead skinny (tongue in cheek moment).

SUMMING UP

There will be setbacks and they will be as different as the people experiencing them.

1   Many visits to the hospital, for many different conditions, did not mean I was in imminent danger.

2   My swollen limbs were dramatically reduced as I worked with a Manual Lymph Drainage (MLD) practitioner.

3   I learnt how to perform MLD on myself.

4   Always look on the bright side of life.

CHAPTER SIX

MASSAGE AND MAKE-UP

Hospital offerings

There is a very sad euphemism in the United Kingdom called the cancer hospital lottery, which means that the quality of care you will receive as a cancer patient will depend on where you live and which hospital you attend. I find this notion unnerving and grossly unfair. I would understand this concept if I was talking about the difference between NHS treatment and treatment which was privately funded. Privately funded hospitals and the way the staff in these hospitals treat their patients is for the most part (like it or not) better and more luxurious when compared to an NHS hospital. The private hospitals have less patients and more money. As the saying goes, 'You do the maths!'

I am not stating that I support this lottery; I am pointing it out because the contents of this chapter are based on the extra support I was given because I was lucky enough to be living in London and to have Dr Faisal Samji as a friend, who booked me into the Royal Marsden Hospital. As their marketing states, The Royal Marsden is a world-leading cancer centre specialising in diagnosis, treatment, care, education and research. So as you can see I was in the top cancer hospital in the United Kingdom. I was being treated within a specialist centre not a general hospital with a cancer ward. There is a world of difference.

Clinical trials

Clinical trials take place all around the country and although I did not know it at the time, I was lucky enough to be invited to join a drug trial. I agreed to take part in the trial because I reasoned that if I only had months left to live I might as well die doing something worthwhile.

Recently I discovered two very important bits of information relating to the participants of drug trials. It seems that they live longer than non-participants. I am not sure where this information comes from, it could just be rumour or legends spread by the trial recruiters or it could be based on an actual clinical trial. I do not know if it is a generic truth; all I do know is that it most certainly was true for me. The second benefit of signing up for a drug trial, which I was also unaware of at the time, is that the participants have more check-ups and if something is not quite as it should be, the participant is quickly attended to. So these are two very worthwhile reasons for joining a drug trial.

It mattered not a jot to me – I joined the trial for purely altruistic reasons and because I had nothing to lose. Now, I will never know if I was on a placebo tablet or on the trial drug and I am not bothered because the results were positive for me. I know there is a belief that you must be stupid if you think a chalk tablet is the real thing, only I also know that the power of the mind to heal the body is phenomenal. I am interested in the outcome, the end result, and if that means life; I really do not care if I have to take chalk tablets every alternative Saturday whilst dancing the tango in my birthday suit. Perhaps my focus on end results was one of the reasons, years later that I was drawn to becoming a life coach.

Massage

Previous to being diagnosed with cancer I was very naive, I thought massage was what prostitutes offered. So imagine my surprise when the hospital offered massage to its cancer patients within a clinical trial. My mother always told us, 'Never look a gift horse in the mouth.' My horsey friends explained that when you go to buy a horse you always look into the mouth as you can determine the age of the horse. Therefore, the meaning of the saying is to just accept it, and don't ask any questions. With this principle in mind, I volunteered for the trial. I was a little bit apprehensive as I had no reference points to guide me, except the prostitute version which I kept forcing to the back of my mind, telling myself that the hospital would not offer massage delivered by prostitutes to its patients.

The day arrived and I made my way through the hospital to the allocated room. It was a new experience and I was deeply moved, which has left such a vivid memory for me. When I entered, the room was lovely and warm, with dimmed lighting and gentle flute music playing in the background. The lady masseuse was dressed in a professional white tunic with a clip board in her hand as she guided me to a chair at the side of the massage couch. She proceeded to do a thorough investigation of my medical history. She asked about the type of cancer I had been diagnosed with and the treatment I had received. Once she had all the information she needed to complete her form she recommended that I have a back massage, which seemed like a good start to me. She asked, 'Can you lie down on your front or will this be too painful for you?'

I was reassured by this question and replied, 'I think it will be too painful to lie on my front because at night if I roll over onto my front I wake up immediately because of the pain.'

This was obviously not a new model of working for her and as I could not lie on my front (breast still very painful).

She asked 'Do you think you can manage leaning against this pillow on to the couch?'

'I am not sure, but let's give it a go and I will tell you if it if becomes too painful,' I answered.

'Yes, please do tell me if you are at any time feeling uncomfortable and I will stop immediately, 'she reassured me.

She asked me to take off my jumper and bra but as I could not wear a bra, I took off my top and gently leaned into a massively soft pillow. She proceeded to warm some base oil and enquired, 'Do you know if you are allergic to lavender oil?'

'I know that I am not allergic to lavender oil as my granny used to rub it onto the bumps and scrapes I would often acquire as a child,' I said.

She warmed her hands by rubbing them together and then she added some oil and started to gently stroke my back. She continued to perform effleurage, (I know this sounds like a very dirty word in the light of the fact that I linked prostitution with massage) but it comes from a French word meaning to touch lightly by using a series of gentle massage strokes when giving a Swedish massage. Without warning, I was overcome with a huge sense of loss. I cried silently, I could not stop myself it just flowed from me. I had no idea that up until this very point, I had hated my body since the operation. I think I felt that my body had let me down. The fact that a stranger could touch my body without being revolted by it moved me beyond myself.

The masseuse did not say anything during the massage and when she had finished and I had dressed I was embarrassed and apologised for crying. She told me that nearly every one of her cancer clients had cried the first time they had received a massage. I was so impressed with the power of massage, I have qualified as a masseuse and now I offer free massage to friends and family if they are suffering from muscular strains or just plain stress related tightness of muscles. I have a massage at least once a month to keep my body supple and calm my mind.

Make-up

Remember back in chapter 2, I told you that every day I would struggle to ensure that I had applied make-up before my visitors arrived. Well, sometime during my hospital stays (I had many, because of complications after the operation and of course the mumps!) I do not remember exactly which stay or what position in my cancer voyage, the nurses came around with bags filled with a variety of make-up from the leading cosmetic companies and gave them to all the women on the ward.

The generosity of the cosmetic companies moved us all. Now I know they write it down against corporation tax and that by giving us gifts we would be predisposed towards their products, should we survive, but it did not matter. Some of the patients on the ward were as poor as church mice and had never paid more than a couple of pounds for any item of make-up, so to get a free bag of expensive make-up was for them, like waking up in heaven. Actually, although I could afford expensive make-up I did not spend very much and it was a great treat for me also.

My cousin was recently diagnosed with breast and lymphatic cancer and she mentioned that the nurses gave her a package full of expensive make-up and she was overjoyed, so it seems that the custom is still happening and I am very pleased about that.

SUMMING UP

I was offered different programmes, trials and goodies during my hospital treatment.

1   I took part in a new drug trial.

2   Massage does not just help to heal the body, it can heal the soul. It can also stop you hating your body and feeling it has let you down.

3   The expensive make-up gifts added to my sense of well-being.

CHAPTER SEVEN

SAYING MY FINAL FAREWELL

Getting ready to die

'Do you think a party is a good idea?' she asked.

'Well Mum, yes I do. The way I look at it is, if I make it to my 40th then I really should celebrate the occasion and if I don't make it, you can still go ahead with the party but call it a memorial event.'

'Oh don't be so morbid, we would not want to party if you have passed over,' she said.

When I was first diagnosed by the young boy in the Gibraltar Hospital and then it was confirmed by the Royal Marsden Hospital, I was given 9 months to live. Having finally become used to this fact I began to think about the end. I know this sounds really depressing and very negative, only I don't remember feeling that way about it. Remember, I had relaxed into the knowledge of cancer and I had a pragmatic approach to it.

Being given the news that I had 9 months left to live, was first announced just before Christmas 1992 and then again in

January 1993 by the Royal Marsden, which happened to be the same year as my 40th birthday. I was born under the sign of Libra in the month of October. I was not sure if I would make my 40th birthday as it was past the deadline. Whoa what a word! I can honestly say I had never considered the extra significance to the time line description. Regardless of the possibility of being dead on the deadline I decided that I would plan a big birthday celebration to be held in the village hall close to where my family were living and where I was born.

Once I had thought about the party it seemed like a great idea and I called my mother to tell her about it.

What is it with phrases like, "passed over", or "passed on"? Sounds like the children's game, pass-the-parcel where, when the music stops (possibly a euphemism for death), the child holding the parcel unwraps it and once the music starts again, the child "passes the parcel" onward to the next child. I suppose when I faced death I was happy to call it by its name and my mother, who did not want to think of me dead, did not want to call it by its name in case the calling of death, brought it on.

'Call it a wake then. Quite why a party for the dead should be called a wake is beyond me,' I said.

'It's called a wake because people used to stay awake by the coffin saying prayers. Not because people wanted the dead person to wake up. Although it could be, if you have a party for the dearly departed, maybe the racket created by the singing and dancing would wake the dead!' Mum has a weird sense of humour and a funny creative mind.

'It doesn't matter what it is called, just continue to have the party even if I don't make it. Remember, I will be watching from the other side and if you don't have the party I will come back and haunt you!' I jokingly threatened.

'Okay dear, if you are sure this is what you want?'

'Yes Mum it really is and I know exactly where I want to hold it. I am going to see if the Bridestowe Village Hall is free, that way all the family can come,' I said triumphantly.

'What about all your friends in London, don't you want them to come?' she said anxiously.

'Don't worry Mum, they love a party and a chance to get a weekend in Devon will add to the attraction. I am sure they will want to come and quite frankly, the ones who think it is too far to come to celebrate my birthday aren't worth a second thought.'

I did not want to tell anyone, but I wanted a party to say goodbye (not literally, just in my mind) to everyone when they would be having fun and I could be silently saying goodbye to each and every one. I wanted to hold the party in Devon because it is the county of my birth and I wanted to invite my old school friends, the old youth club members and most of my family, who lived in the West Country.

I booked the village hall and I also booked Molly, the best caterer for miles around. I ordered two large birthday cakes and arranged for an outside bar for the drinks. Then I spent weeks sending out invitations. Now I know that sounds as if I had thousands of friends – it took weeks because I was up and down with my energy levels due to the treatment. However, because I did invite everyone I liked and as I had studied, lived and worked in many different places with many different groups of people, there were a fair few people to invite.

It was during this period that I received my goodies bag from the cosmetic companies I mentioned in the Make-up and Massage chapter. I loved the make-up and it started me thinking about having a raffle at the party to raise money for research into reducing cancer. I contacted all the cosmetic companies who had donated goodies for the Royal Marsden Hospital bags. I explained what I wanted to do and asked them if they would donate a gift box of their products for my raffle. Every single one agreed and they sent me beautiful large gift boxes which were cellophane wrapped so people could see what was inside.

Then I had a thought: if these companies are willing to give gifts for raffles, which other companies might be willing to promote their products via a raffle? In the end I managed to get 30+ extraordinary prizes for the raffle. There were so many prizes it took two trestle tables to display them and 35 minutes to do the raffle at the party!

I thought long and hard about the music, as there would be a mix of young and old people, country folk and Londoners, farmers and fashionistas, postmen and programmers, hairdressers and handymen, doctors and nurses, bankers and bakers and everyone in-between. I decided to book a country band often called a Ceilidh band; only they play country songs. The band is made up of musical players and a "caller". It is the caller's job to teach the partygoers each dance by getting them to practise the dance before the band would strike up. Once the dancers have run through the moves the band plays the tune which accompanies the dance and the caller then calls out the moves as the dance progresses to lead the dancers. I thought this would be perfect as everyone would be at roughly the same stupid level of competency and would therefore have loads of laughs as mistakes were made.

My cousin, Phil Down, is in a Barbershop band which to the uninitiated is a group of four singers each with his own vocal part, using harmony to create the sound. As this was going to be my secret goodbye party I asked Phil if I wrote some notes about special people in my life would his band be able to make up a song about them. He said yes they would and so it was arranged that midway during the party when the country band was resting and the food was served Phil's Barbershop Band would sing the song. It was a great success and went down really well as I had selected the most bizarre, funny or outrageous things the important people in my life had done, which not only made them laugh, the rest of the partygoers also found it funny. The party was great fun and it was lovely to see people from my school days and youth club days having as much pleasure as the London set.

On reflection, and we all know that hindsight is a great thing, I think all the activity and planning to organise the party was a great distraction from the radiotherapy which was taking place. Consistently thinking about a happy event instead of the negative side of the treatment, as I later discovered when I started learning about visualisation and affirmations, could have helped me to cope and possibly influenced in a small way the extending of my life. You will find that I did a lot of little things towards healing; I am a very strong believer in the power of compounding the little things.

I guess by now you are wondering how much money the raffle raised. Well I don't really know for sure because at the end of the party we had two people at the door rattling boxes and demanding all the loose coins in pockets or purses be put into the boxes which also added to the funds.

On top of these two fund raisers I had put in the birthday party invitations that I did not want any presents (I thought I would have no need for anything with such a short life span ahead) and I would be happy for cash to be put into a cancer charity birthday jar or if they wanted to give cheques, could they please make them out a cancer charity of their choice or the Royal Marsden Cancer Charity. That evening my family and friends raised nearly £3000 for cancer charities (approximate equivalent value in 2016 of £5,500) and we all had a fantastic evening as well. I was so proud of them, especially as the majority of the partygoers came from low income households. If you were one of the partygoers and are reading this, thank you from the bottom of my heart for your generosity.

After the party I wrote to all the companies who had generously donated gifts for my raffle and told them how much we had raised for cancer charities, not separating out the raffle from the other activities as I decided that would be inconsequential and diminish their generosity. I wanted to encourage them to continue giving gifts to fund raisers.

SUMMING UP

Saying goodbye whilst having a fun filled party was a great way to live!

1 Distraction is a great tactic; thinking and organising a fun filled event was a great distraction.

2 Fundraising was good for my soul and for my healing.

CHAPTER EIGHT

FORGIVENESS CAN SAVE YOUR LIFE

When you let go of hurt and truly forgive, you set yourself free

Remember, way back in chapter one I told you about Pete's (my boyfriend) response to the cancer. He said, 'I cannot deal with your cancer. I think we should go our separate ways.'

Well after my crying storm, I decided not to spoil our Christmas so I said to Pete, 'I think we should make the most of Christmas and then when you drive me to the airport after Boxing Day we can go our separate ways. What do you think?'

'Yes, okay, that seems fine to me,' he said.

So we did the best we could during the couple of days we had together and when it was time, he drove me to the airport in my car. He was staying in Spain until New Year's Day and I let him have the use of my car during this period. When we had arrived at Malaga airport, I said 'Thanks for driving me to the airport, please remember to put the car keys in the sideboard drawer when you leave. I wish you all the best.'

'Uh, we will see each other again,' he said as a statement of fact.

'No. We will not be seeing each other again. We agreed that we would spend Christmas together and make the most of it and we would finish our relationship when I left to go back to the UK. You were the one who said you could not deal with this,' I pointed out.

'Well I think I have changed my mind,' he said

'It's too late for that now. I have come to terms with coping on my own and I do not want you in my life anymore nor do I want you contacting me again, as I need all my concentration on the cancer,' I said in a calm and centred way. I could not forgive him for the cruel way he handled things and I did not want someone who reacted in this way in my life.

'Don't be like that,' he implored.

'I have to go now.' I kissed him on the cheek and promptly left him as I rushed through the departures gate.

Forgiving Pete

I cannot remember much about the time between when I arrived in the UK and New Year's Eve as it was filled with hospital visits and settling in at Faisal's. I can however, remember some of what took place on the evening of New Year's Eve. My cousin, Keith Down, came to see me and I drank myself into oblivion, whilst moaning to him about the vagaries of life and cancer. I remember being very sick in the bathroom toilet. I ended up with a massive hangover to start the New Year and I suppose this was how the rest of the year passed for me, like a massive hangover without the pre-drinking fun.

Faisal popped his head into my bedroom at some point on New Year's Day to tell me he was going out and that Pete had telephoned to say he was going to come and see me. I felt so sick and nauseated I told Faisal I would not be answering the door and he need not worry.

Later that day I had started to feel hungry and hungover so I made my way down to the kitchen to rummage around for something to eat when the doorbell rang. I had completely forgotten Faisal's words of warning and I staggered to the door. On opening the door I remembered but it was too late, there stood Pete with a hangdog expression on his face, 'Hi, can we talk?' he asked.

'No, go away,' I replied in a very quiet voice as speaking aloud sent pains through my head.

'I want to talk to you and I am not taking no for an answer,' he stated in a very stern Royal Marine Sergeant Major voice which sounded like Big Ben's chimes were residing in my head. I could not deal with the situation so I just left the door open and shuffled back into the kitchen. He followed me and proceeded to batter me into submission with words of regret and requests for a second chance. I think he was cleverly taking advantage of my hangover because I caved in and I said that if he wanted to hang around he could. He did hang around and eventually I forgave him. He is still hanging around to this day because I found that by forgiving him I allowed our relationship to grow and I eventually married him! Forgiving can have some amazing results.

Forgiving my body

Now here is a different story about forgiving which involves a visit to a masseuse. A big part of the healing process for me came after a massage where I discovered that I hated my body because it had let me down. It was an illuminating moment but one that, at the time, I did not know what to do about or how to move forward from this revelation in a positive way. Everything started to come together during the manual lymph drainage massages I discussed in the Setbacks chapter. I had learnt how to perform the MLD massage on myself and this required that I stroked my body many times a day in a gentle soft way. The subtlety of the massage's effect on changing my body loathing into body loving was miraculous. It is difficult, if not impossible, to be gently stroking your body and at the same time hating your body, the action and emotion being too incongruent for the unconscious mind to reconcile – something had to go! I was determined never to suffer the pain of lymphedema again, so the massage stayed and the hate seeped away.

As you know, I forgave my past during the weeping and wailing on the first night. I forgave Pete; the forgiving started slowly and ended in a marriage. And this is a marriage which has not only given me a partner for life it has also given me the space to write the Coaching Handbook Series, other books on coaching and this book. I have forgiven my body through the introduction of massage. These different forms of forgiveness were not done as a conscious activity. I did not say to myself, 'I forgive you.' The process was natural and wonderful. The thing is I was trained as a teacher and once a teacher, always a teacher, which means, if something happens to me or in my life which has a positive learning, I have a deep burning desire to be able to replicate the learning and then teach it.

I do not know when or even who introduced me to *The Dynamic Laws of Prosperity* by Catherine Ponder, however I do know that she has some perfect sayings (incantations) for conscious forgiveness. Now before you worry that I am about to go all religious on you, I am an atheist. I am also very curious and have a thirst for knowledge which enables or creates the environment for personal growth. Not forgiving someone is the antithesis of this and creates an environment for loathing where healing of any kind has great difficulty. To be able to read her book I had to mentally replace the word God with Universe and once I did this, I found a world of very useful incantations. Here is a powerful forgiveness incantation adapted from her book – the blank underscored space is the name of the person to forgive.

_____ I fully and freely forgive you. I loose you and let you go. So far as I am concerned, that incident between us is finished forever. I do not wish to hurt you. I wish you no harm. I am free and you are free and all is again well between us.

If you repeat this often enough you will start to believe it and eventually you will be able to say the incantation free of negativity and what is more, you will actually mean every word you say. As soon as I notice that I am not struggling to say the incantation, it is my way of knowing that forgiveness has taken place deep within me.

At first, I found this little incantation a huge challenge, however there were equally huge rewards. Chanting this incantation when all I really want to do is poke the other person's eyes out with a hot poker is a huge challenge, I have to admit. Trust me and stick with it because the reward of letting go of the negativity is worth the effort of the challenge.

Forgiveness was a big part of my healing process. The thing is – not only did I have to deal with the cancer and forgiving, I also had to deal with the way people behaved around me because I had cancer. Some avoided me completely, acting as if the cancer was highly contagious. Others spoke in hushed voice with exaggerated sympathy and some just treated me the same as before. Initially, I resented the first two categories of response until I eventually realised that they were the ones with the problem and in due course I found a way to forgive them, which set me free from negative energies.

SUMMING UP

In my model of the world, healing takes place after for-giveness has started.

1   I had to learn to forgive my body.

2   I forgave Pete and the rewards for this forgiveness come every day of our married life together.

3   Forgiving friends brings a multitude of different joys.

CHAPTER NINE

CAREER SETBACKS

A setback was a catalyst to a completely new life and career

At the start of Chapter 5 'Setbacks', I said that setbacks were only stumbling blocks on my road to recovery; here the setback was the dawning of a new life. Once I had forgiven Pete and our relationship had developed, we agreed that I should move out of London. After pooling our resources we bought a house in Bournemouth, which was close to Pete's place of work. The major draw for me was the closeness of the sea. I have always found the sea to provide solace and a space for healing to take place so it was a perfect move for me.

Preparing for an interview

Having moved to Bournemouth I needed to find employment. I applied for several jobs, all of which I was suitably qualified for plus I had the experience and competencies for the roles. I have always been successful at interviews because I would take the time to learn about the company, its vision and mission statements, the names and details of the directors. I would prepare my experiences to match the job specification and I rehearsed my answers to questions thus ensuring I would come across as knowledgeable and interested. I prepared questions I wanted to ask, because asking interesting questions continues to build on the picture of a suitable candidate for the role. I think only once in my career prior to cancer, had I been unsuccessful in securing a job from an interview. I could go on a long time about this – in fact I've written a book! It's *The Personal Success Handbook*. Check out Chapter 11 'Interview Success', if you want all of my tips and hints for effective interviews.

I attended my first interview and was, as I expected, offered the job. As I was leaving the interview room the manager asked, 'Just before you go, we have a Private Health insurance programme for all our employees, and I just want to know that you will pass a health check won't you? You haven't any serious illnesses we should know about?'

'Well I have just recovered from cancer and I am healthy so it should be fine,' I replied cheerily.

I went home on cloud nine; I had a new job, new home and a lovely partner to share my home with. I excitedly told Pete all about the interview and how I had been offered the job.

The next morning at 9.30am the phone rang and it was one of the interviewers from the day before. After introducing herself she said, 'We are terribly sorry to tell you but there has been a company reshuffle and the job is no longer available. We wish you success in finding another position.'

Just like that! Bam! No job. I had my suspicions that it was the news about the cancer that had killed the job offer but I could not be sure at that time. After six more job offers and six more changes of decision once cancer had been mentioned I was completely despondent, distraught and depressed. I had rarely taken a day off work in my long and successful career and had no intentions of letting the cancer affect my new roles, if only someone would give me a chance. They would not!

Fortune favours the brave

Scrutinising the local paper for any job, I saw an advert for a freelance computer trainer for a local training company and I sent in my curriculum vitae. I did not want to work for myself; I was scared of being self-employed as I had always been a model employee.

Weeks went by and I had just started to apply for cleaning jobs having decided not to reveal the cancer even if it was lying by omission. I needed the work; I had a mortgage to pay. One Wednesday morning the phone rang and this very bubbly lady said, 'My name is Angela Brown and I run a computer training company. You applied for the freelance vacancy a few weeks back and I wondered if you were still available?'

'Yes I am,' I replied.

'Well I am sorry for the delay in responding only we had a work experience school pupil working in the office and she put your application in a drawer and I did not see it. Can you come in later this morning for a chat?' she asked.

'I would love to. Let me take down your address, I can be with you in about 50 minutes. Is that any good?' I had calculated the time it would take me to put on a suit, make-up and get into the town centre. We agreed the time and she explained the way to reach the office. Once I put the phone down I thought, 'Why did I say yes?' and this would not be the only time I would ask myself this question.

After the interview she said she would love to have me as one of her contractors and she had a job for me the following Monday.

'That will be lovely, what was it?' I enquired.

'It is a 2 and ½ day Microsoft Word course. We usually run them back to back so you will be working all week. The first course will finish at 12.00 Wednesday and the next course will start 1.00pm. You will have just enough time to clean down the computers and reset the room,' she announced.

I felt nausea mounting as I responded, 'I have never used Microsoft Word, and I will not be able to take this job. I am happy to learn it for a future job.' I had yet again lost a job, this time not because of the cancer but because I did not know a bit of software.

'Don't be so daft. You have taught Wang's Word Processing software for years, so learning Microsoft will be easy for you and besides I am in a hole and you would be helping me out of it,' she said.

I was not so convinced it would be as easy as she made it sound, 'But I don't have a laptop to practise on.'

'No problem, I will lend you a laptop and you can take the training manuals home with you. Look, it is my biggest client. The training is in the head office of a global bank and I have been let down by one of my contractors. If I cannot find a trainer for Monday I will lose the contract and it's a contract to supply all the Microsoft end user training for their head office. I would go myself only I am already committed to a training contract where the client has specified the trainer has to be me. Please say you will do it? I promise you that if you have problems or do not understand something you can call me. I will teach you over the phone or you can come into the office. If you have problems during the training I will talk you through it over the phone.'

On reflection this was the perfect scenario for me – someone in trouble that I could help and I had no time to worry about being self-employed. I am a very fast learner and many times during my years with Wang Laboratories I had to train on the job. It involved teaching a topic and whilst the delegates were practising the skill just taught, I would be learning the next topic ready to deliver it with confidence and not a small bit of acting.

I left her office with a laptop under my arm, computer manuals in a carrier bag, her business card in my handbag and a big wave of fear crashing over me. 'Why did I say yes?' I asked. I spent all my waking hours before Monday learning how the laptop worked and then how the Microsoft Word software worked to a very basic level of understanding. It was very different from the Wang Laboratories Word Processing, although the underlying principles were the same.

Monday morning arrived after a very bad night's sleep. I put on my best suit and my shoes were polished to a mirror like shine. I arrived at the bank's training centre and eventually found the training room. There were 12 PCs (personal computers) and none of them were turned on. I started to feel panic rising and I asked myself, 'Why did I say yes?' I cannot say what number of times I had asked myself this question since I had first met Angela Brown.

I had arrived early so I thought I had plenty of time only when I turned on all the computers, I discovered that the software exercises for the course I was delivering had not been loaded as I had been promised. Luckily, I had been trained well at Wang Laboratories to always expect the unexpected, so I had copied the exercise files from the loaned laptop onto a floppy disc. (For the uninitiated, floppy discs predated CDs as a form of computer data storage.) I hurriedly loaded all the exercises needed for the course to take place, 12 times on to each individual computer and I was just finishing as the first couple of delegates arrived. By now I was sweating and red in the face! I slapped on the Wang Smile (as we used to call it, smiling whilst panicking) and the day got off to a scary rollercoaster of a ride. I survived the first course and was an expert by Wednesday lunchtime ready for course number two. The start of self-employment had arrived for me.

Being turned down for those jobs as a direct result of having cancer was the best thing that could have happened. If I had found an office job I would never have experienced the thrill of working for myself. Come to that, I would not have become a bestselling author nor would I have the pleasure and privilege of coaching, training and mentoring so many outstanding people. Cancer was the catalyst for this wonderful change in my career direction. The setback of being turned down for so many jobs could have proved catastrophic for me but instead those setbacks put me into the position of being desperate enough to risk my career and plunge headlong into self-employment.

SUMMING UP

Every cloud has a silver lining and the cancer cloud is no exception.

1 Changing career is not always a bad thing.

2 Being bold and brave has its rewards.

3 Stepping outside of my comfort zone was the beginning of a completely new way of life.

CHAPTER TEN

KNOW YOUR ENEMY

Knowledge is power

Firstly, let me be clear that it is not good to think of cancer as your enemy. I thought long and hard about the title of this chapter, as I wanted to attract the attention of readers who "Fight Cancer." I want to challenge this approach where cancer is seen as the enemy. I did not think I was fighting cancer as I had an intrinsic wisdom that the energy required to wage a war would be exhausting and this energy could be better re-directed towards healing. I admit at the beginning I did not like my body and I hated the cancer, which is quite different to waging war. Now if you feel that waging war on your cancer is right for you, it is your decision and your body. There is however, another way to succeed.

New feel

In the last chapter I mentioned working as a self-employed trainer, and once I had settled into the new role I decided I wanted to train as a masseuse because it had made such a difference to how I felt about my body and cancer. I found an ITEC Swedish Massage course in Ringwood which was taught on a Sunday over several weeks. It was perfect for me because being on a Sunday it meant that I did not miss any opportunities for self-employed work during the working week. I was very nervous on the first day of the course but I did not need to be as there were only three of us and although the trainer was a real stickler for details and was strict, the other two women on the course were fabulous and we had great fun.

This course required lots of study of the body, not just structural and muscular; we had to learn about skin, cells, lymph, blood, heart etc... We also had to learn the contra indications of massage and on top of all this theory we also had to find 30 clients to practise on!

I passed the course and although I did not set up a massage practice the information I learnt on the course has been invaluable. The other wonderful thing about the course was that it started me thinking about cancer cells. I researched cancer, the lymphatic system and white blood cells, lymphocytes and phagocytes. I discovered these are the cells that protect the body. I also learned that the phagocytes ingest foreign particles, bacteria, and dead or dying cells. I found pictures of phagocytes (pronounced phage o sites) and pictures of cancer cells from the many books I had purchased for the massage course and I memorised their form.

Now, this was a long time ago and these days I cannot be sure if I had already learnt about visualisation or not. I just remember very clearly what I did. Every night before I went to sleep and every time I went to the toilet (I have since learnt this is called visualisation with anchoring – the process, not the toilet!) I would conjure up my phagocytes in pairs. I had re-named them Faggo sites as it made me smile. I imagined a double castle gate opening and the Faggo sites pouring out in pairs by the hundreds. Then I would picture the cancer mass being eaten on all sides by the pairs of hungry Faggo sites. Each time I did this I would see the cancer mass getting smaller.

I would send these Faggo sites off several times a day and last thing at night. Now who knows what effect they had on my recovery and more importantly, on preventing the cancer from continuing to metastasize? I am not actually able to specifically say the visualisation impacted on my recovery. Only that all the little things I did and still do, when added together and compounded have given me 23 extra years of an outstanding life. I am still counting the years.

Food for thought

During the studies I learnt about food and the effects of food on the body, which started me off on the study of food and nutrition and the links with cancer. This is a fascinating topic and many books have been written by far wiser people than myself on the topic. I will share with you some of the changes I made to my diet, with some of the results, and you can decide what's right for you.

I became a pescatarian, not vegan nor a vegetarian. The name, pescatarian, where does it come from and what does it mean? Well Wikipedia spells pescatarian differently, (with an e instead of an a), and says that a pescetarian is probably a neologism (apparently this means a new word has been made, where the user has a distaste for it) which has been formed as a blend of the Italian word pesce "fish" and the English word "vegetarian". I eat no meat – that's it. I eat fish, dairy, carbohydrates, everything (not any foods I do not like the taste of) except meat. Coming from a farming family I take a lot of teasing about not eating meat and that is fine by me. I feel better for it and that is what counts.

I was given a book about a doctor called William Howard Hay, who became ill with Bright's disease, inflammation of the kidneys, which he could not cure with the medicine of his time. He realised that we are what we eat and being clever, he spent time thinking of how the stomach digests food. Some foods need an acid environment; some foods need an alkaline environment, to enable the food to be broken down for digestion to take place. Then he thought that when you mix acid and alkaline you get a neutral PH environment which is not the best condition for food to be digested and it also produced unwanted waste materials. He created a way of eating called food combining, or the Hay diet, where you only eat food which requires the same environment for perfect digestion. All acid or all alkaline, plus foods he considered to be neutral which can be eaten with either. He cured himself and went on to write many books on the subject. I followed the Hay diet for many years and I am not too far from it in my current food consumption.

Initially, I went into changing my diet considerably and passionately and now I have settled into what suits me whilst still being considered healthy. I bought a juicer and only purchased organic fruit and vegetables but I soon tired of cleaning the juicer and gave up on that pursuit. I also tried green wheatgrass juice but I could not be bothered with it all. So instead I just eat loads of fruit, vegetables, nuts and fish. I had heard raw beetroot was considered a good cancer preventative food in Russia; I ate a lot of beetroot, raw and cooked, and I still do.

Food fear

Thinking about the saying "you are what you eat" gives me a nervous feeling in the pit of my stomach which has nothing to do with the food I have eaten. I have just talked about how I changed my diet after all the research I was doing. I was concentrating on eating to help my body heal itself. What really impacted me happened when I expanded the thoughts about eating for a future me to encompass my eating habits from the past. What caused the nervous stomach is the knowledge that I might (the jury is still out on this) have eaten my way towards cancer. If it is true, that we are what we eat, then on this thinking trajectory it will follow that my previous eating regimes must have had an impact on the growth of the cancer or at the very least, created an environment where cancer could grow! This is so profound that it makes me feel helpless when I think about prevention of cancer through diet.

Before cancer I was a massive coffee drinker, having about 10+ cups a day which I completely stopped for many years and now I have a couple of cups in the morning and hot or cold water the rest of the day. I had not partaken of any alcohol (except the odd glass of champagne) since I was 22 years old. The reason I gave up alcohol was because I went on a real bender (massive consumption of alcohol one Sunday night) and had to go to work the next morning. I had a great pal staying with me and she also had to go to work the next day. We crept out of the house (creeping was the quietest form of movement with the least jarring on the head) and we gently kissed each other goodbye. She was going left from the front door and I was going right. I remember turning around to see if she was okay when a dizzy sickness came over me and I am ashamed to say, I was sick in a neighbour's garden.

I stood up, wiped my face and continued on to work. I said to myself on that morning 'I will not drink alcohol again.' and it was as if my body agreed with me because from that moment on, if I took a drink of alcohol (except champagne) I would instantly develop a cracking headache, which felt like someone had put a metal band around my head and was tightening it.

Anyone who knows me now will be saying 'hang on a minute, when I was having dinner with Curly the other night she was drinking wine!' They could also say, 'What about New Year's Eve after she had arrived back from Spain? She said she was drunk then?' Correct. Let me explain.

After my chemotherapy I went to a wedding with Faisal and I had not had anything to drink since breakfast. The wedding was one of those long drawn out affairs when the photography took longer than the wedding ceremony. The problem was that the bride and groom had forgotten to provide any liquid refreshments for their guests in-between the wedding and the wedding breakfast. I knew, through experience, that non-alcohol drinkers do not get served a drink until way after the wine has been poured, if at all. I have been to many events where I have had to make several requests from the serving staff for a non-alcoholic drink and even getting a glass of water can be a challenge. I said to Faisal, 'I am so very thirsty, if

I take a drink of wine and I get a reaction, do you have anything in your bag (meaning doctor's bag) to counteract it?'

'Yes, I do,' he replied.

I gulped down a glass of wine and waited. Nothing happened. I was amazed and having since chatted with Faisal about this, we guessed the changes to my body from the chemotherapy could be the cause of the non-reaction. Every cloud has a silver lining.

New Year's Eve 1992, I imbibed enough champagne to have a shallow bath in. The point here is that I only had the occasional glass of champagne (holidays, weddings, special events) prior to my diagnosis. With this logic (nor sure if it is logical) alcohol played no part in the growth of my cancer as I did not drink regularly nor did I drink heavily (excluding New Year's Eve 1992 by which time cancer had arrived).

Besides the change to my diet, I had read somewhere that the current mass produced foods did not contain sufficient vitamins and minerals. I started to take a daily dose of multi-vitamins, one thousand milligram of vitamin C and 50mcg Selenium, and I still do. I know there is a school of thought (can you imagine a school solely filled with thoughts, what a great place that would be – well only if they were happy positive thoughts) that taking vitamins and minerals is wasted because most of the intake is expelled by the body and you can/should get them all from a varied diet. I am not prepared to take that risk and if I only had money for vitamins and minerals or a new dress, the dress would not be purchased. If there is a small uptake of goodness from the tablets, that small uptake could be the difference in outstanding health and good health. Remember what I said about small things compounded producing big results.

SUMMING UP

I went on training courses and read lots of books on the human body and cancer.

1   I used energy and visualisation to heal myself instead of fighting my body.

2   No comment on alcohol as not enough experience to be able to judge.

3   "You are what you eat" therefore what I have eaten has created me as I am now.

4   Supplements are just that.

CHAPTER ELEVEN

CANCER OF THOUGHTS

Negative thoughts will affect the healing of the body

What you think about will be what you get or, as I put it in The Personal Success Handbook, "A thought attracts a corresponding positive or negative experience." This leads to the concept that what you think about is what you will experience, an idea that has been popular among certain philosophers and denominational devotees for centuries. There is a famous reference said to be from Gautama, also known as Sakyamuni, the key figure in Buddhism, which suggests that, what you have become is the result of what you have thought. The followers of the Law of Attraction have used this quote as a form of proof to support this theory along with a Jewish proverb, "As a man thinketh in his heart, so he is." They also claim that quantum physics backs the theory which arouses my curiosity.

Looking back over my life prior to cancer I can clearly see the signs and the thought patterns which may have contributed to the cancer growth. The first and very clear negative thought pattern I can remember was during a seven year relationship I had back in my twenties. The guy wanted to make money. It was his main driver and money for him equalled success. To earn the money for him to invest in a rundown property, we both worked during the day as employees and again every evening. We would put on our overalls and paint and decorate flats around London for a builder friend. Having worked the evenings, we were then even booked to paint and decorate a two bedroomed flat, in one weekend; and then a different flat every weekend! We would get up with the sparrows, drive to the flat and work until the job was done. I packed the food and drink as well as doing the painting and decorating. I was lucky to get 4 or 5 hours sleep a night. We continued this pattern of double jobbing until we had enough money for a deposit on a rundown house.

Once we had the deposit for the house, we continued working in the day jobs, followed by spending our evenings and weekends doing up the house we lived in. There were months of no hot running water, I would have to carry buckets upstairs to use the toilet, which incidentally you could see from the floor below as most of the floor boards had been removed. To wash, I would boil water in a saucepan and strip wash in the kitchen. Once a week, we would go around to his mother's house for a bath. I remember as clearly as if it was last night that every night during this period of my life, as I dropped off to sleep, I would ask the universe not to wake me in the morning. I would say, 'Please do not wake me, pass me by and wake others instead.' Wow, this is such a bad thing to ask for!

Just as soon as the house was completed, he decided he did not love me anymore. He had found someone else. I was mortified, crushed and heartbroken. On reflection, I had sacrificed myself for him by neglecting myself. All my money and my time I gave to creating his dream and because I did not invest in my clothes, self-esteem, beauty regime, entertainment and joy of life, having taken what he could from me, he then found the rest in someone who was not exhausted and who spent time and money on herself! That was a lesson I learnt the hard way.

Abandonment and rejection

His abandonment and rejection hit me hard and in those days I knew nothing of self-development and positive thinking, so I drowned myself in negativity for many years. On the surface I looked like a successful business woman with a vibrant and varied social life. When home alone in my apartment, I would be filled with self-loathing. I hated my body (I thought I was too fat at a size 12!) and I was unhappy with my life. I spent huge amounts of time and energy over many years thinking negative thoughts about myself and, as is often the case in people dissatisfied with their lot, I also held negative thoughts about others. I had all the trappings of materialistic success but I always felt there was something missing in my life. Had I spent the time reading self-development books and attending motivational seminars (I am not sure if there were many around in those days, to be fair) I think my cancer would have had difficulty growing in a body full of positive energy.

Here is what, if I had known at the time, might have prevented my cancer developing or at least, restrained its growth. If I had known before cancer, about the impact of beliefs, the power of self-talk and how we create the rules of life, I would have enjoyed the success and I would have loved my body as I do today.

Beliefs and self-talk

For me, the beliefs and self-talk cycle go hand in hand so I will cover both together. I am going to use a simple example so that you understand how it all works. When I was younger my family liked to play tennis and I remember we would go to the Cornish resort of Bude, where they had lovely grass tennis courts which overlooked the sea. We would hire a court for a couple of hours and play tennis. I was not very good at it and although I was spending time with my family I was always on the losing side of the net. I developed a belief about my abilities as a tennis player; I would say to myself, 'I am a lousy tennis player.' This is a definitive belief about my abilities because I used the words, 'I am' meaning it is true and in the present time frame.

My family helped with this belief because they would say, 'You are useless at tennis,' or other similar encouraging comments. So I told myself I was not good at tennis, others told me I was no good at tennis and when I would go to play tennis, with all this proof, my body would support me by not putting the ball where I wanted it to go. As I would hit the ball in the wrong direction or miss it completely, I would say to myself, 'I am a lousy tennis player,' and my partner in the doubles match would also be saying something similar. Whenever I thought about playing tennis I would picture the missed shots, my serves outside the boundaries and I would hear my internal and the external commentaries.

I had created a loop of my self-image (seeing myself missing shots); followed by my self-talk (I am a lousy tennis player), which created the missed shots. Once I had missed the shot I would repeat the self-talk, 'I am a lousy tennis player' which would re-inforce my negative self-image of my tennis abilities. This, I later learned, is a self-talk cycle. Interestingly, I carried this belief for decades until I started to wear contact lenses. I have astigmatism and this meant for me that when I wore the contact lenses I could see exactly where the ball was. When I did not wear the lenses, there was a gap between the position of the ball and where I saw it! I was not a lousy tennis player after all but the self-talk cycle kept the limiting belief alive.

This example of a limiting belief has not really affected my life much. Only one of my boyfriends liked tennis and he would not have liked to be beaten at the game by me. The thing is, I had many other controlling limiting beliefs which crushed my life, my relationships, my happiness and my success. The most common one was believing that I was not worthy of ___, the blank can be filled with almost everything I entered into. One of the great things about contracting cancer is learning all this stuff; there is no rule that you have to have cancer to learn it though. (See rules below.)

Knowing all about how beliefs are created and held within a self-talk cycle is liberating. I now know how to spot a limiting belief, how to change the words into a positive statement about myself and thereby create a new belief which is positive and supports my successful happy life. How liberating is that?

Rules

I have to be honest before I start on this topic – I had more rules than you could shake a stick at. What am I thinking when I make this statement? Well, we all have things that have to be in place before we can be something or someone. We often want things in place before we can do something. Let me explain this with an example of a question I asked myself:

"How many things do I need to have in place before I can say I am happy?"

The staggering answer to this question was 'many'. Most of us decide that many things have to happen (sometimes in a special sequence) before we believe we are happy, successful, loved, healthy, or whatever. Here are only a few of the things I used to believe needed to be in place before I could say I was happy.

> I had to be half a stone (3.18 kilos) lighter
> I must have a boyfriend who is handsome
> I had to have £30,000 cash in my bank account
> I must be loved unconditionally
> I had to be wearing designer clothes
> I must be a success (I had other rules about what had to be in place to be a success)
> I had to be invited to the "in" parties/first nights
> Etc…

I know now that all of the above items on my list are irrational and unreasonable.

I think I learnt about the rules of life from Anthony Robbins, but I cannot be sure as it was more than 20 years ago. Whoever it was, I thank them from the bottom of my heart because learning about the rules of life has set me free. I learnt to fully accept myself (be happy). To do this I had to realise I was the one making my rules and worse, I was the one ensuring I obeyed them. Think about this now for a few minutes. I set myself ridiculous rules which all had to be in place before I would LET myself feel happy and then I ensured I kept to this bizarre new ruling. Okay, before you start pointing the finger at me and saying what a stupid fool I was to let this happen, I want you to ask yourself the same question and answer it honestly. You will have to think about this very hard as it is easy to be self-delusional when you first start examining your own rules.

Knowing about rules gave me permission (I did not actually need permission – another set of rules) to be happy for any reason whatsoever and here are a few easy to obtain rules about happiness straight off the top of my head. I have also used the "I am _____" to create a core belief about happiness at the same time.

> I am happy whenever I wake up in the morning (this is a great one)
> I am happy whenever it rains
> I am happy whenever the sun is up
> I am happy whenever a stranger says 'Hi'
> I am happy whenever I see a cat
> I am happy whenever I make a stranger smile
> I am happy whenever I listen to music
> I am happy whenever I breathe
> I am happy whenever I am alone
> I am happy whenever I am in company

The list is, and should, be endless if you want to live a happy life in your model of the world. Now here is something I avoid, adding "because" followed by a reason. The more you have to have reasons for being happy you are backing up an underlying rule. Sounds complicated, however it is easy if you allow it to be easy and it may help if you remember that there are no rules except you keeping them and there is no need to have a reason for changing the rules.

Once I had understood this simple and effective approach I started to look at all the things that affected me. I examined the rules underpinning the way I behaved and what I believed to be true. I am totally responsible for making my life difficult by my responses to circumstances and I can make my life easy if I choose a different response. I make the rules; I can break them. Yippee!

Every so often, I find an old set of rules controlling the way I respond. I forget that I am in control. Sometimes I forget I am the driver of my own bus of life. Only the difference now is I can recognise my self-imposed restrictions and I choose to change them.

SUMMING UP

I am in control, I take responsibility, I enjoy the changes I make and I set myself free.

1   I am what I think about most of the time.

2   I liberated myself from myself.

3   I have healthy, happy thoughts.

4   I make my rules, this means I can break them.

CHAPTER TWELVE

MUSHROOMS AND OJIBWAY INDIANS

This is beyond alternative therapies and only for the brave

I need you to open your mind as wide as it will go and then a little wider because I am going to tell you about some "out there" stuff which I tried. Let's face it – I had nothing to lose. So I had a go at a few things and I enjoyed stepping outside my comfort zone into a weird world. I want you to remember that modern medicine or conventional medicine as we know it, has not been around long (since approximately 1800) and when I compare it to natural remedies, which have been around for centuries, it was a no brainer for me to evaluate some of the alternative cures and potions available.

Some of our commonly used modern medicine has its roots in nature. The humble aspirin, for example, has its origins as far back as Hippocrates, who left records of using ground up willow bark and leaves to treat headaches, pains and fevers. Willow bark and the leaves produce a chemical

n as salicin and it is this chemical which gives willow
its therapeutic effects. Specialists believe that the chem-
alicin, when processed by the body, transforms itself
salicylic acid, which is the chemical precursor to aspirin.

Essiac Tea

Therefore, in my model of the world it made sense to give
some of the nature based remedies a go. I am going to start
with Essiac tea because I really feel it made a difference. I
used it for two years and would use it again in a heartbeat.
I heard about this remedy from an alternative health practitioner who gave me a leaflet explaining the origins of the tea.
I loved the story behind the remedy. Very briefly, a Canadian
nurse, Rene M. Caisse was working with terminal cancer
patients where she met a woman who claimed to have cured
herself of breast cancer from a formula she obtained from an
Ojibway Indian. Nurse Caisse obtained the composition of
the formula and prepared some. She started giving the tea
to her terminally ill patients, with the permission of their
doctors, getting great results.

The main herbs in the mixture are burdock root, slippery
elm bark, sheep sorrel and Indian rhubarb root. Rene named
the mixture Essiac which is her surname reversed. Her story
is very interesting, only I do not want to risk prosecution by
writing about it and there are many websites dedicated to
telling the story and offering the herbs either dried or made
up into the tea ready to drink.

I first bought the readymade tea and then I decided to make
my own. It is a fiddly business involving boiling, seeping, muslin
and sterilised bottles. It gave me something active to do towards

my healing and I think that taking part in the healing process not only gave me something to do, it also acted as a thought changer. Being part of my own healing in a physical and mental capacity made a difference. Back to the tea, it tastes disgusting and I am of the "old school of medicine", by which I mean, as my mother would say, 'If it tastes awful it must be doing you some good!' Quite how she came to this conclusion is way beyond my understanding and way beyond my courage to challenge her. Thus, as is the way with family sayings, I continue with the belief, daft I know, and I moderate the saying with the circumstances. For example, I would not take or imbibe a known poison such as arsenic no matter what the taste.

Here is the bit you need to know to keep me safe from prosecution – no extensive clinical studies have been performed as yet which would provide conclusive evidence that Rene M. Caisse's herbal formula/mixture will alleviate, cure or prevent any disease or condition.

There are many websites with further information and whilst you are on the internet have a good look around for others. Wikipedia puts a contrasting side of the story of Essiac tea and I recommend doing research and comparisons to give you a balanced view.

Now as you have read this far in the chapter you may be thinking that I was "game for anything". I will temper that statement; I was game for anything related to a possibility, no matter how remote, of helping my body heal itself.

Kombuca Tea

As drinking tea seemed to be high on the list of things to do I heard of another type of tea, Kombuca tea, which, I was told, is made by fermenting a symbiotic colony of bacteria and yeast. "SCOBY" is another name for it and is an acronym for "symbiotic culture of bacteria and yeast." Mushroom to the likes of you and me, although I have been admonished many times for calling it a mushroom! I like to poke fun at people who I call stuffed shirts and I just cannot help myself.

This Kombuca mushroom, not to be confused with the magic mushrooms, although I had heard they are a lot of fun, I bought off the internet. The SCOBY duly arrived with instructions on how to make it in a jar. I decided I wanted to make a batch, so used a plastic bucket! I do not recommend this method. I made up the bucket with a mixture of tea (normal breakfast variety) and sugar then put the mushroom or SCOBY into the bucket and covered the bucket with a muslin cloth. I put the bucket in our spare room to ferment.

The day after, I was offered a couple of large training contracts and I promptly forgot about my tea making venture. Our spare bedroom at that time was south facing and lovely and warm. I came back home after being away on one of the work contracts to find Pete looking a bit perplexed. He said, 'You know that mushroom stuff you made up a while back?'

'Oh my God, yes. What has happened?' I asked in a nervously anxious voice.

'I think you should go to the spare bedroom and see for yourself. It stinks mind you,' he added.

I put down my suitcase and rushed up the stairs. As I opened the spare room door the smell of a slightly sweet and sour brewery tickled, no, slapped the back of my nostrils.

'Wow. It stinks in here!' I said as I turned to Pete, who wanted to see my reaction.

'You haven't seen it yet!' he pointed to the other side of the spare bed.

The bucket could not be seen. Where the bucket should have been was an enormous fungus which had covered the bucket and was now edging its way towards the door. I think it was planning to take over the world, starting with our carpet.

'What do you want to do with it?' Pete enquired, in a weary of your experiments, kind of voice.

'Get rid of it,' I said as visions of Triffids and the like came to mind. I could see myself being smothered whilst I slept by a slightly damp and slithery mushroom. This was not the way I had planned to die. Pete painstakingly extricated the mushroom from the carpet and bucket and put the offending SCOBY in the bin. So I have nothing to say about this tea that will be of any benefit to anyone, except, if you do decide to make it, remember to look in on it every day and start with a very small batch!

Marijuana

Marijuana, also known as C or cannabis, is a plant which has been used for medicinal purposes for over 3,000 years they say (who they are, I am not quite sure!). Cannabis is classified (as I go to print) in the B drug group in the UK. The American, National Cancer Institute has very interesting things to say about cannabis and cancer. I was told that cannabis relieved some of the symptoms associated with cancer and I would have considered sourcing some except I had already been introduced to it.

A few years prior to my cancer diagnosis, I shared a flat in Shoot Up Hill (I loved the address) with a girl called Maria (name has been changed) and she had a boyfriend who liked to smoke the weed. I had never considered it as, to be honest, I am much too much of a control freak to want to give up my faculties to some mind enhancing drug. I was fairly pompous at the time, which I have mentioned before. I used to smoke "normal" by which I mean legally supplied cigarettes, about 20 a day habit. Maria and her boyfriend had been badgering me for a long time to give it a try and to judge for myself. One wet Sunday afternoon, I went around to their flat. They were both high and I was bored. I said I would try a smoke. We shared a joint and I felt very sick. They were giggling as I left to return to my own flat where I was sick and promptly took myself to bed. I woke up the following morning which was of course a Monday morning with a headache compounded by the Monday morning blues. I think that says enough to explain my reticence in using or smoking the drug marijuana.

I decided without fanfare that I would never touch the stuff again and even cancer could not tempt me into going back on my word. I have however, heard that many cancer sufferers have used cannabis to great pain relieving effect and many also swear by the pain respite marijuana offers.

Colonic irrigation

Colonic irrigation and coffee enema are two things I have considered, but to my shame (I could not open my mind wide enough or my legs) I was too pathetic to experience this form of remedy or treatment. I am still sitting on the fence (I thought that phrase would amuse you) on this issue and I may one day give them both a go. If I do I will write a blog about my experience, until then, I recommend you research colonic irrigation and decide for yourself. Bottoms up!

SUMMING UP

I looked into many different alternative remedies/treatments, some of which are described in this chapter.

1   Having an open mind was a critical factor in my healing.

2   Essiac tea from the Ojibway Indian formula I think helped my recovery.

3   Kombuca tea is not a mushroom it is a SCOBY.

4   Cannabis made me sick years before the cancer.

CHAPTER THIRTEEN

RACE FOR MY LIFE

Two stone to lose

When I was moaning to Faisal (remember him from chapter 1) about the cancer, he said that the bright side of having cancer and the treatment that goes with it, was that I would lose weight. Every cloud has a silver lining, but Faisal's prophesy was totally incorrect in my case. I know that it is common knowledge in the oncology world that weight loss is normal during the treatment for cancer. Only for me, I became two stone (12.7kg) heavier with a puffy face, lymph-edema in my arms and I had grown three times in my dress size: I had been a UK dress size 12, now I was wearing UK dress size 18 and I looked like a whale in clothing. So much for the bright side of life!

Exercise

I was living with a sinewy ex Royal Marine (he says there is no such thing as an ex Royal Marine. Once a Royal Marine always a Royal Marine) who considered exercise the same as breathing or eating. He could not understand why I was dismayed at his suggestion of my taking up running as a form of exercise. Eventually, he convinced me to join a gym which I started going to and the gym physical trainer designed a programme especially made up for the fat lady. It started off with a gentle introduction to the gym and its myriad of machines which all looked like torture mechanisms to me. I can say that having used some of them I think they are torture mechanisms.

Gym was not the answer

It was early in the year and for some strange reason I kept getting colds or flu. Contracting colds and flu was very unusual for me as I had been looking after my health in a very conscious way due to the lowering of my immune system from the cancer treatments. I just thought it was because I was mixing more with people and this increased mingling with strangers increased my likelihood of picking up viruses and bacteria. One day I was able to go to the gym around 11.00am and I was in the gym on my own. I was using this machine where you sit down (perfect for me) look at a screen and cycle in a near sleeping position. I was bored so I looked around and this fit looking guy had entered the gym and he started his routine on the treadmill. As he was running he kept coughing and blowing his nose into his hand towel. That put me off him to be truthful! I thought, you should not be in the gym if you have a cold, it cannot be good for you. As the treadmill slowed down to a stop he took the hand towel he had been blowing his runny nose into and wiped down the machine! I never returned to the gym and I never will.

In this vulnerable state, Pete convinced me that getting out in the fresh air and running would be much better for me and that I needed a goal (the seeds of coaching were being planted). So I entered the Bournemouth 5k Race for Life. It was one of the best things I have done; I had a goal, I had a personal trainer (sergeant major), and I could train by running on the promenade and looking at the sea. What could be better? Okay, some of my friends might say 'sitting in a deck chair with a glass of wine in my hand looking at the sea' would be better! I was truly blessed, I lived by the sea, I lived with my love and I worked for myself which meant I could go for a run whenever I wanted. I loved jogging first thing in the morning when everything was fresh and crisp and the sea smelt sharp and full of life.

Jogging and chanting

Have you seen the American Armed Forces jogging in formation all chanting to a rhythm,

'Dah duh, dah duh, dah dah dah

Dah duh, dah duh, dah dah dah'

I am not sure what words they use; I just remember the tune and the fact that it matches the beat of your feet as you run. With this in mind I decided to use the chanting for some healing mantras. I had heard of Louise Hay's saying about getting better every day in every way and I thought this would be a great mantra to chant as I jogged. I used to say, 'I get heathier every day, I get healthier in every way.' My chant fitted perfectly with the rhythm of the American Armed Forces chant. Then I became very creative with my chanting adding new varieties. Here is one I remember, 'I get richer every day, I get richer in every way.' It was great fun adding new chants as I jogged along healing my body and my mind. Two for the price of one!

Now let's get something really clear here, it was not my intention to win the Race for Life nor was it my intention to keep beating personal bests. I just wanted to lose a bit of weight and get fit. I had to put my foot down (not a running term) with my personal trainer, and remind him I was not one of his new recruits. Once he realised I would keep up the fitness and I started watching my food intake he was fairly happy. He would occasionally chip in with a running technique and one that I loved to hear about is a fartlek (I kid you not!). The first time I heard this term I was convinced he said 'fart leg' and for a while that is what I thought it was called. It made sense to me; I often broke wind when I ran. Here is a word of warning, do not run down wind of me, in all senses of the words. Apparently, for those of you who are not familiar with training terms this means (from a chillaxed ladies point of view) mixing it up. Running fast and then running slowly, apparently doing this will improve your fitness and speed.

I can honestly say that the jogging really helped me to get back my figure and it helped me to get back my self-esteem. I had not realised that all the extra weight and the large sized clothes had diminished my love of self. Getting heathy was my goal, yet I had not included exercise into the equation. I am now a little older and jogging is too hard on my knees, so every day I walk for 60 to 90 minutes. The difference in time is due to meeting lovely neighbours and 'chewing the cud' (a West Country saying meaning have a chat with them) for a couple of minutes, which enhances the walk. Research now states that a brisk walk (to me it means getting a wiggle on) for 20 minutes a day is great for keeping fit. So get out there and chat with your neighbours.

Dancing

Also, during the initial stages of looking for some form of exercise to do because attending a gym was now out of the question, I remembered I loved to dance. The trouble was that the disco scene where I used to dance had moved on to different music and different moves. What to do instead? I saw an advert for salsa dance lessons and convinced Pete and our dear friends the Edmondsons to join up. Who would have thought that learning to dance could be such fun and quite so complicated? Actually, being a teacher, I am sure it was the training we received not our abilities. I would say that now wouldn't I? The problem was that every week we were taught a new dance without reference to the one we had learnt the previous week. By the end of the term the whole class (except a couple who had been salsa dancing before) were hopelessly confused and disheartened. I could not cajole Pete and the Edmondsons to return for a further term.

When Pete and I moved to our current house in a small and vibrant village, I saw an advert for Scottish dancing classes. You would have thought I had learnt my lessons about competencies from the salsa dancing experience but I am not one to be easily dissuaded. I rang the contact and he sounded very jolly, saying that all levels were welcome. He also mentioned that they danced for a bit then had a cup of tea with biscuits followed by a bit more dancing. It sounded perfect and although we struggled a bit at the start we love going. We have fun, exercise and get to know our neighbours all at the same time. There are no experts or teacher. We just muddle through; find a new dance and all of us work out how we think it is meant to be danced. Lots of laughs and mistakes later and we usually manage to do a reasonable version.

Exercise is important for full recovery and for maintenance of health. I tried the conventional gym membership and it was definitely not for me. What it did was open my mind to alternative ways of keeping fit and healthy which made exercise a happily anticipated activity rather than a chore. I strongly believe that keeping fit must be enjoyed to become enduring.

Deodorants or antiperspirants

Normally when we exercise we perspire and this seems as good a place as any to talk about deodorant and cancer. During my research into cancer I came across articles on the Internet and in the wider press which contained warnings that underarm deodorants or antiperspirants were linked to causing breast cancer. The articles either commented on the aluminium-based compound active ingredient of antiperspirants or parabens the preservatives in some deodorants.

The aluminium compounds work by creating a temporary block to stop sweat escaping. It has been claimed by these various articles, the compound could be absorbed by the nearby breast tissue and cause an oestrogen effect (growth of breast cancer cells) and thus the link to cancer forming cells. The parabens are used as a preservative in deodorants and they have been found in samples of breast tumours. The possibility (however remote) of cancer and the use of deodorant is sufficient for me to stop using them. I no longer use any deodorants or antiperspirants on a daily basis. There are some good alternative aluminium and paraben free underarm preparations available which I use on special occasions (weddings, parties, etc...). I do not want to be called Smelly Nelly by my endearing family members.

Drink more water

The other benefit of exercise is that I had to increase my fluid intake and I would drink water during or just after exercising and then drink buckets of milky tea. Eventually my weight loss plateaued and I was not sure what was going on. I did not fancy increasing my exercise, so I looked at what I was doing besides exercising. I realised that I was drinking 8 to 10 cups of semi-skimmed milky tea a day and someone recommended I try skimmed milk. Yuk! This presented me with a dilemma, what should I do? I started to drink coffee which I can enjoy black and because I did not want to overload my body with caffeine I decided I would try drinking just plain boiled water. The first cup of hot water was a bit weird and now after a couple of cups of coffee, I only drink water, hot or cold. If I am in a café no matter what time of day, I only drink hot water because the standard of coffee or tea in a café can vary greatly and water is nearly always the same once boiled.

Scientist state our bodies are made up of between 60% to 80% water which means a large part of my body is liquid. As I exercise I lose fluid via sweating which I think we all know happens but most people do not know that liquid loss is a natural function of the skin throughout the day. This means we need to drink often to replace this fluid loss in order for us to function. I wanted to increase my intake of water and needed something to inspire me to this. I found a beautiful blue glass bottle and with a little more searching I found a half pint glass (237 millilitres) made of blue glass. With this on my desk I am encouraged to drink more water. I heard from an acolyte of Ho'oponopono that if you put the blue bottled water in the sunshine (quite difficult in the West Country as the sun is rarer than blue glass), the water is energised. I like that thought and I am encouraged to drink more as a result of this.

I am briefly going to mention something I came across during my journey to health regarding water experiments and a Japanese man called Doctor Emoto Masaru. He believed that water could react to positive thoughts and words, and negative thoughts and words. He published *Messages from Water,* which contained photographs of ice crystals which he claimed proved his theories. I love the ideas he expressed, only he did not follow scientific protocol and his experiments have been disputed by the scientific community.

All I have to say at this point is 'Drink Up.'

SUMMING UP

Exercise is important for full recovery and for maintenance of health.

1 I realised that keeping fit must be enjoyed to become enduring.

2 The gym was not the answer for me.

3 Dancing can be a fun way to get fit.

4 Drinking water is essential to well-being and I found different ways to introduce water drinking into my daily routine.

5 Ho'oponopono is an ancient Hawaiian practice of reconciliation and forgiveness.

CHAPTER FOURTEEN

LIGHT AND LAUGHTER

Laugh and the world laughs with you

Funny thing meditation – it seems to me you can either do it or, like me, your inner voice will not shut up no matter what. I really believe we need to have quiet moments and to this end I have been to meditation classes and groups, only to come out feeling frustrated and tense. I get meditation, I really do, and I love hypnosis (when I am taking other people through it). The problem is my inner voice. I have been told that practise will help, only when I sit and start the routine things start to go awry. There are meditation apps which are available and many people find them very helpful, not me.

Alternative meditation

I used to worry about my lack of controlling my inner voice (not a good platform to launch meditation from) and I would feel a failure. Nowadays, I am more philosophical about it. How did I manage this? Being an outstanding coach I looked at my desired outcome and realised it was calmness, joy, peace and being at one with the universe. I get all of these in abundance when I go for my daily walk around the lovely West Country lanes. I spend the time in nature, full of gratitude and overflowing with the joy of life. The rhythm of my walk and the wonder of my experience are truly spiritual. The seasons bring daily changes to the same hedgerows and each corner reveals another of the universe's wonders. I spend the time thanking firstly my body and then everything else.

Neuro Linguistic Programming (NLP)

I realise this sounds like some computer lingo and it also can appear very complicated. It is not about computers and in my model of the world (an NLP description of how I experience the world) I thought it was easy to understand and very practical in its application. In 1994 I booked myself on an introduction to Neuro Linguistic Programming course. NLP has been described as the art and science of personal excellence. I have written about NLP before in *The Life Coaching Handbook, everything you need to be an effective life coach*. I understand NLP to be a series of techniques and procedures for coding human behaviour to assist the understanding of what people do and how they do it, when they perform with excellence. John Grinder and Richard Bandler were the founders and their work was built on studies and observations of three excellent therapists: Virginia Satir, Milton H. Erickson and Fritz Perls.

Back to the NLP practitioner course I had enrolled in. It was mandatory that I attend a four day introduction course beforehand and I had missed that year's introduction course by two days. The company was generous and gave me a 1-to-1 introduction course with the amazing Dave Marshall in order that I could attend the practitioner's course. Dave Marshall was the lead trainer on the NLP course and he was outstanding in every way. Almost all I know about NLP, and I know loads, comes from his training. I think he worked on the principle that if the student wanted more and demonstrated understanding, he would continue to teach.

During one of the sessions he gave me a Representational Systems Preference Test. It involved my selecting different responses to situations under a stressful time focused condition. After completing the test he gave me something else to do whilst he marked the test. When he returned he said, 'I am astounded, I have never had a result like this. Your preference is auditory, only your score on auditory is nearly maximum. You only have small scores on the other preferences.' To put this in context I will need to cover a little bit of NLP here and rather than re-inventing the wheel I will quote from my book, *The Life Coaching Handbook:*

When an external event happens to us, we run our own perception of that event through internal processing. We create our own 'Navigational Chart of the Sea of Events' that depends on the way we prefer to remember things. We store and remember events by making an internal representation through our senses. The predominant senses we use during these storage and retrieval processes are visual, auditory and kinaesthetic. To a smaller extent, the olfactory (smell) and taste senses are also used, but their impact is not significant enough to be examined here.

Although you use all of your senses, all of the time, there are occasions when you use one sense predominately.

When listening to a music concert on the radio you would principally be using your auditory sense. If you were having a shower, you would be predominantly accessing your kinaesthetic sense, as you would be feeling the sensation of the warm water caressing your body. If you visited an art gallery, your primary visual sense would be used.

Dave was amazed because I seemed to use only, or mostly, auditory to interpret the world. He asked me to create a picture in my mind. I did not understand what he meant. It was an absolute revelation to me that people created pictures in their heads. He helped me to construct some pictures, which was a weird experience for me. He explained that to be an excellent communicator I needed to develop my visual and kinaesthetic processing and language skills.

Getting back to meditation, I have a theory that people with high auditory preferences find it hard to quieten the inner voice because it is the inner voice through which they experience the outer world. If I experience things through my auditory sense and my inner voice, I could not experience a meditative state because I would have to turn off the means by which I experience it, thus I cannot experience it. Seems to make some sense to me, but then it would as I have a high auditory representation system. I am, as I write this book, listening to Sir Van Morrison's music; his music has been with me through all my book writings. Although I can write when there is silence I am only prolific when there is Van Morrison. When I was younger I could only study with music in the background and I would spend all day singing.

So I gave up on traditional meditation and replaced it with my own route to inner peace and abundance. I have a process I follow to take me there and in that respect the procedure is similar to meditation techniques I have tried. In meditations I was taught to follow my breathing then work up or down my body relaxing each part of my body to get to ... who knows where, I never got there.

The process I use is a step by step gratitude process. I thank every part of my body in turn by saying,

'I love you my _____ thank you for protecting yourself, healing yourself and keeping yourself healthy and healed.' I do this for every part of my body. When I have completed my body I look around and thank everything individually as I see it. I then thank the universe. There are always moments of overwhelming joy during my walks. Who needs class A or B drugs when you can achieve euphoria by being grateful whilst surrounded by nature?

I learnt some of the above process from Dr. Joe Vitale and Dr. Ihaleakala Hew Len, from their book *Zero Limits*. They tell a true story of the unusual therapist who helped heal an entire ward of mentally ill criminals – without seeing any of them. Ric Hayman, a very dear friend of mine, told me about the book and I am truly grateful to him. The book introduced me to Ho'oponopono (mentioned in the last chapter) which is an ancient Hawaiian practice of reconciliation and forgiveness. Dr. Hew Len tells us we are responsible for everything in our lives and we can use repentance, forgiveness, gratitude and love as the forces to cleanse the unconscious mind of data, which will allow us to get to zero, a place of creation. This is not a good description of Ho'oponopono and if you are interested I recommend further study. Dr. Hew Len has many videos on YouTube which might help. Meditation and/or finding spiritual solace creates a space for healing to take place.

Laughter

Now along with meditation I looked at laughter healing, only I don't think it had a name back then. I did realise that I felt a whole lot better after a good belly laugh (and as you know from previous chapters, I have a good belly). During my chemotherapy and radiotherapy there were days when I felt so low, emotionally and physically, that I found it hard to do simple tasks and I just lay on the sofa all day. It was on days like these that I would put on a funny movie or listen to a humorous audiobook or comedy CD. I realised I always felt better afterwards but I did not at the time know it was a form of healing.

I believe I first heard about laughter as a form of healing around 1994 from Joseph McClendon III on a Tony Robbins seminar which I attended and I have already mentioned earlier in the book. Joseph was a platform speaker on the last day. He told a story about his mother and how he took a television into her hospital room, along with some videos of funny programmes for her to watch because laughter has healing powers. I have always looked on the funny side of life and I love to make people laugh. I hope you have had a few giggles already whilst reading this book? On returning from the seminar, and being curious, I started to investigate the impact laughter has on the body. Here is an extract from one of the books I have written in the Coaching Handbook Series, *The Personal Success Handbook, everything you need to be successful:*

When we laugh, our bodies produce T-cells, Gamma-interferon and B-cells all of which produce disease and infection destroying antibodies. Laughter stimulates the release of the body's natural painkillers called endorphins. This all amounts to a general sense of well-being and can speed up recovery.

I could not think of a more fun way to aid my recovery and so proceeded to read funny books, watch my favourite comedians and attend the theatre to see comedy plays.

When we laugh we activate the limbic system to produce endorphins which in turn create a general feeling of well-being similar to taking opiates. Opiates are derived from opium (poppy plant) and they are a group of drugs used for treating pain with close links to codeine, morphine and heroin. The word opioid is used for a whole class of drugs including synthetic opiates. The point I am making is, laughter can produce a similar sense of well-being to taking drugs.

This endorphin production can also happen during exercise. People who exercise to continuously reach a new personal best will often take themselves past their physical limit – they call this hitting "the wall" which can become the driver for the exercise. When they hit the wall, they feel a sudden rush of euphoria (endorphin blast) which enables them to overcome pain and continue exercising.

Sexual addiction can also be explained; the endorphins produced during sexual intercourse become the addiction and the person loses the normal moral guidelines in order to satisfy the need for the euphoric experience. Another endorphin stimulant is eating chocolate (or drinking hot chocolate) as this is known to increase the levels of endorphins, serotonin and phenyl ethylamine (also known as phenylethylamine), being released into the brain and thus increasing the feeling of well-being.

The main healing process for me where endorphins were involved was laughter and sometimes the odd bit of chocolate. Remember that all the little steps towards healing, when compounded, create a swell of healing and health.

SUMMING UP

Meditation and/or finding spiritual solace can create a space for healing to take place. Laughter produces endorphins which aid well-being and in turn healing.

1   I was unable to meditate and replaced this with spiritual walks.

2   Spiritual space is also said to aid recovery.

3   Laughter releases endorphins which can have a pain relief effect and creates a feeling of well-being, so I watched funny films and listened to comedy programmes.

CHAPTER FIFTEEN

MUSEUM OF OLD BELIEFS

NLP and the Museum of Old Beliefs

As I have briefly mentioned in previous chapters, during my search for a cure I came across NLP (Neuro Linguistic Programming) which seems to me to be an umbrella term for lots of good stuff. Within the umbrella are therapeutic interventions, powerful linguistic techniques, deep level communication and future pacing. Let me break NLP down into simpler terms. Neuro (neurology) relates to how our bodies function, Linguistic covers the way we communicate with each other and Programming is all about the way we behave. So as you can see NLP seems to cover all the aspects which have, or could have, an impact on the growth of cancer.

This is the reasoning behind why I have dedicated a chapter to one of the powerful interventions which can easily be performed at home with little or no NLP background. You can work through the process with a friend and you do not have to have cancer for this powerful technique to work for you. This simple process can be used to change any negative belief (a belief can be defined as any thought you consistently have about yourself). You can, for example, work on a belief about your body, your confidence, your skills or competencies. I have given you an example below and as you work your way through the technique you will see that you can use it for any negative belief you have. Here is an idea: you can ask a friend to walk through the process with you and then you can walk him/her through one of their negative beliefs. This way you both benefit.

As the title suggests, I am going to talk about an intervention called the Museum of Old Beliefs, which was developed by Robert Dilts. I did not train with Robert Dilts, so I am not sure how close my version will be with his original ideas. The adaptation I was trained to use is so easy to follow and yet it can offer profound changes. I think one of the advantages of NLP is that the practitioner/therapist does not have to know the content or details of the client's limiting belief; this means that you can work through very personal stuff at a deep level without the practitioner knowing what you are working on. All the practitioner needs to know is that you are working on something. In my model of the world, the skill of an outstanding NLP Practitioner is intensive observation coupled with responsive, gentle guidance. In the example below I include content so you can clearly see how it all works.

Briefly, the process involves the client identifying a limiting belief they wish to rid themselves of. The client is then taken on a journey where they visit an old museum and leave the belief in a trunk in the attic of the museum. Sounds simple; the thing is there are some horrible things that can go wrong if you do not set the intervention up properly with a safe anchor. I am going to go through the whole set up as I was taught it using the old belief 'I have cancer'.

Practitioner: 'Have you identified the belief you wish to replace?'

Me: 'Yes, thank you.'

Practitioner: 'Do you want to share it or would you prefer just to give it a name we can both work with?'

Me: 'I am ok to share this with you. The belief I wish to work on today is I have cancer.'

Practitioner: 'Is that what you want to call it?'

Me: 'Yes.'

Practitioner: 'What do you want to replace this old belief with?'

Me: 'Well, um, I am healed and healthy.'

Practitioner: 'Here are four pieces of A4 paper: Safe Place, Old Belief, Museum of Old Beliefs and New Belief. Please can you place them on the floor with the Safe Place on your left, the Old Belief immediately in front of you, the Museum of Old Beliefs a couple of steps in front of the Old Belief sheet followed by the New Belief a couple of steps ahead of that.'

Me: (I place the sheets as requested.)

Practitioner: 'Okay, I am going to set up the safe place and then we are going to create the new belief. Please stand next to the Safe Place sheet. I want you to think of a time in your life you felt perfectly safe. It can be when you were a child, when you are at home or wherever. (Pause) Have you remembered a safe time?'

Me: 'Yes, it was when I was in my hay bale den on the farm I grew up on.'

Practitioner: 'That is good, did you feel really safe in your den?'

Me: 'Yes, absolutely.'

Practitioner: 'Okay, tell me about your den, what did it look like?'

Me: 'Well, it was like an igloo in as much as I had to crawl into it. It smelt of fresh grass and I had a blanket and pillow where I would lie down and just spend time.'

Practitioner: 'Imagine you are in your hay den now.' (Watching for subtle changes in body and facial language.)

Me: 'Yes, I am there.'

Practitioner: 'Now I want you to increase the smell of the fresh grass, feel the blanket and pillow and tell me when you feel perfectly safe by saying "I am safe" and as you say "I am safe" I want you to step on to the Safe Place sheet.'

Me: (after fully remembering the experience of being in the den) 'I am safe.'

I step onto the sheet as I feel her hand on my elbow. (This is anchoring, another NLP technique described in *The Life Coaching Handbook*.)

Practitioner: 'Please step off the sheet.'

Me: 'Okay.'

Practitioner: 'What did you have for breakfast this morning?' (Asking a non-related question during an intervention is known as breaking state.)

Me: (thinking this is weird) 'Uh, porridge.'

Practitioner: 'That sounds good. Now I want you to step back onto the Safe Place sheet and at the same time take yourself back to your den.'

Me: 'Okay.'

Practitioner: (checks to see that my facial and body language are the same as when I stood on the safe place last time. Sees that I look the same.)

Practitioner: 'How safe do you feel?'

Me: 'Very.'

Practitioner: 'That is fine. We are now ready to create the new belief. Please can you move to just in front of the New Belief sheet? Imagine you are healed and healthy.' (Pauses.)

Me: 'Yes okay.'

Practitioner: 'How do you know this to be absolutely true?'

Me: 'Well, I am in the oncologist's office and she is hugging me as she says you are healed and healthy.'

Practitioner: 'Look around you, what do you see?'

Me: 'I see the posters of the human body on the walls, a tree outside of the window, the sun is shining and she and Pete are smiling.'

Practitioner: 'What are you feeling?'

Me: 'I am bursting with happiness.'

Practitioner: 'What are you saying?'

Me: 'I am healed and healthy.'

Practitioner: 'Step onto the New Belief sheet now please.' (As I step onto the sheet she places her hand on my shoulder.)

Practitioner: 'Please step off the sheet now. What did you have for dinner last night?'

Me: (thinking, what is this with food) 'I had vegetable fajitas.'

Practitioner: 'I am now going to take you through the process and I want you to follow my instructions and when you have completed each task, simply say one word – "there" to tell me you have completed the task.'

Me: 'Okay.'

Practitioner: 'Please stand on the Old Belief sheet.'

Me: 'Okay.'

Practitioner: 'What is your old belief?'

Me: 'I have cancer.'

Practitioner: 'Now I want you to imagine you are walking down a cobbled street in an old part of town.'

Me: 'There.'

Practitioner: 'Step off the Old Belief sheet as you look around the street and notice all the old shop fronts and the people walking by with their heads down. It is raining.'

Me: 'There.'

Practitioner: 'As you are walking along you see a sign on the left and it says Museum of Old Beliefs. There are steps up to the museum and the big ornate wooden double doors are open. You walk into a large foyer with a big crystal chandelier in the centre of the ceiling.'

Me: 'There.'

Practitioner: 'On your left is a small open door leading to a stone spiral staircase. There is an arrow pointing the way. You start to walk up the stairway.'

Me: 'There.'

Practitioner: 'You keep on going up and up and round and round.'

Me: 'There.'

Practitioner: 'Then suddenly you find yourself on a small landing. In front of you is a door with a sign on it which says "this door can only be opened with a key" which you will find in your left pocket.'

Me: 'There.'

Practitioner: 'Have you found the key in your left pocket?'

Me: 'Yes.'

Practitioner: 'Open the door.'

Me: 'There.'

Practitioner: 'You are standing at the open door of the attic room. At the far end of the room you can see a wooden box with your name on it. You walk to the box and open the hinged lid.'

Me: 'There.'

Practitioner: 'You discover you are holding the old belief in your left hand. Put it into the box and shut the lid.'

Me: 'There.'

Practitioner: 'You find that you have another key this time in your right pocket which locks the box. Lock the box now.'

Me: 'There.'

Practitioner: 'When, and only when, you are completely sure without doubt that the old belief is locked in the box you leave the room and close the door behind you.' (Pause)

Me: 'There.'

Practitioner: 'Lock the door now.'

Me: 'There.'

Practitioner: 'Make your way down the stairs and at the bottom of the staircase turn right and go out of the museum doors. As you walk down the steps you hear the museum doors slamming closed and the sound of locks clicking into place.'

Me: 'There.'

Practitioner: 'You walk down the street and out of the town up to the top of the hill which overlooks the town. When you look back at the town you see the Museum of Old Beliefs is alight.'

Me: 'There.'

Practitioner: 'You stand and watch as the museum burns to the ground and everything in it becomes ashes.'

Me: 'There.'

Practitioner: 'When you are ready and only when you know in your soul that your old belief has been destroyed and no longer exists, step off the sheet.' (Pause)

Me: 'There.'

Practitioner: 'Step on to your New Belief and remember the oncologist's office. See the tree through the window, see the poster of the human body on the wall, the sun is shining and she is hugging you, Pete is smiling. You are bursting with happiness.'

Me: 'There.'

Practitioner: 'Say aloud, I am healed and healthy.'

Me: 'I am healed and healthy.'

Practitioner: 'On a scale of 1 to 100 percent bursting with happiness, where are you?'

Me: '80%.'

Practitioner: 'We are going to take this up to 100%. Now I want you to turn up your feelings of bursting with happiness, make the colours sharper and the smiles wider and shout out loud, I am healed and healthy.'

Me: 'I am healed and healthy.'

Practitioner: 'Again and louder.'

Me: 'I AM HEALED AND HEALTHY.'

Practitioner: 'On a scale of 1 to 100 percent bursting with happiness knowing that you are healed and heathy, where are you?'

Me: '100%.'

Practitioner: 'Again and louder shout out, I am healed and healthy.'

Me: 'I AM HEALED AND HEALTHY! I AM HEALED AND HEALTHY! I AM HEALED AND HEALTHY!'

Practitioner: 'Well done! I want you to repeat this mantra and as you do, remember the bursting with happiness feeling for a minimum of 50 times a day which is easy to do. Only five separate times a day, saying I am healed and healthy, for 10 repeats.'

End of intervention

Now, there is no guarantee that this worked; what I do know is that I still say 'I am healed and healthy' every day. I also say 'I am happy, healthy, wealthy, wise, healed and whole.' The Museum of Old Beliefs can be used for any limiting belief and I have used it hundreds of times with my coaching clients.

I have even used it over Skype for non-critical limiting beliefs. I ask my client to set the camera in a place where I can see all the positions and then see how she/he responds to the first part of the exercise, the setting up of the safe place. If this works well, I will go ahead with the whole process. Only once have I stopped the process and advised the client to find a local master NLP practitioner to take them through the procedure. The underlying driver for all my coaching, is that I always work in the client's model of the world and I am always doing what is right for the client, not what will keep me in control of the client.

Remember, if you feel a bit daunted by the process and would still like to go through it, I suggest you do a search for NLP master practitioners online. Select one who uses the Museum of Old Beliefs intervention and whom you feel you like the sound of.

SUMMING UP

There are many interventions under the NLP banner and the Museum of Old Beliefs is a powerful one which I like to use because it is relatively simple and at the same time produces profound changes.

CHAPTER SIXTEEN

MERCURY MATTERS IN TEETH

Mercury poisoning from dental amalgam fillings

I realise talking about teeth and amalgam fillings seems very remote from our topic of cancer but I have proved, and I completely believe, that the path to healing for me involved lots of little things which on their own seem almost irrelevant and when added together over time complete the healing picture. Hence a chapter all about mercury in amalgam fillings.

If you do not like going to the dentist I suggest you skip this chapter as it is all about dental work. Only, if you have a lot of black/grey fillings in your mouth I suggest you stick with it as there are some interesting findings here for everyone.

Somewhere, someone mentioned that amalgam fillings in teeth contain mercury which seeps into the mouth continuously. If your fillings are old, the release of mercury is higher. Well, I thought, let's have a look in my mouth. Wow, about 80% of my teeth had amalgam fillings! I started to investigate and found a group of people saying that there was no need to worry about the amalgam fillings. This group of people consisted mostly of dentists. Another group of people were saying that the amalgam fillings should be removed immediately as mercury is very toxic. Mercury naturally occurs on our planet and it is said to be the most poisonous, non-radioactive substance. This sentence alone should be sufficient for anyone to ask questions about the long term effect on health of having a mouth full of mercury based fillings.

Apparently, since the 1970s (I was in my twenties at that time) the amalgam filling used has a high copper non-gamma 2 level (I have no idea what this means) which releases a lot more mercury (the important bit) than the previous type of amalgam filling. And the fillings are thought not to be as stable. What this means is that the fillings break down more quickly and mercury can escape. Because our cheeks and under the tongue easily absorb mercury it can get into the body quickly and into the lymphatic system and blood. Once this happens it is like having a free bus pass to all the routes around the body as lymph and blood are everywhere.

'How does mercury poisoning present itself?' was my very first question, and I bet you are thinking the same. There is a very long list of symptoms so I will just cover the headline ones to give you an overview.

Mercury is said to affect the central nervous system and the symptoms seem a little vague (I do not mean that the symptom is vague, I mean the linking of symptom with mercury). Mercury has been classified as a neurotoxin which could be related to irritability, restlessness and mood swings which are some of the symptoms; I must have had a bucket load of mercury in my system as at the time, all of those symptoms fitted. I also suffered from lethargy, drowsiness and insomnia all of which could be mercury poisoning, or the effects of a pressurised job.

There are obvious oral symptoms such as a metallic taste in the mouth, bleeding gums and ulcers. Again I could put my hand up for all of these. Gastrointestinal problems are stated as side effects. I had been a long term sufferer of irritable bowel syndrome (IBS) which I had put down to the stress of the job I was doing before I was diagnosed with cancer. Could the IBS be related to the mercury in my system?

The list for systemic symptoms is long and again vague: headaches, allergies, skin problems and loss of weight (I was not affected by loss of weight). There are also cardiovascular effects which I am happy to say I did not suffer.

The problem with discovering the symptoms of mercury poisoning or any other illness is that I am inclined to find at least one of the symptoms which match what I have, or I have had in the past.

After lots of research and debate with myself and my friends, I decided that I would have my amalgam fillings removed and replaced with resin composite fillings. Some dental scientists considered the risk of mercury poisoning from amalgam fillings was very low or non-existent and I had included this information in my decision making process.

The process to replace the amalgam fillings with composite fillings sounds simple; it is not simple. I had to find a dentist who could and would do the work and who also understood the reasons behind the extractions. I needed a dentist who would minimise my mercury exposure during the removal of the amalgam because the removal of amalgam fillings can disperse mercury vapour. If the patient is not properly protected during the process, there is the possibility of swallowing mercury. I did not want to swallow mercury in any form.

I found a lovely dentist who fully understood my concerns and he had already performed the procedure several times. He allowed me to speak to previous patients where he had removed the amalgam fillings. After all the research, I was ready to go ahead. This is not a cheap procedure and I weighed the costs of the removal against possible harm to my body from seeping mercury. I weighed up the release of mercury from the procedure and finally decided that the short term risk of amalgam removal outweighed the long term health impact of retaining them. I also considered the fact, as told to me by this dentist, that resin composite fillings do not last as long as amalgam fillings and were prone to falling out or breaking down.

There was another factor which had to be taken into account; amalgam fillings are dark grey and quite ugly. When I laughed all anyone saw was a wall of dark grey amalgam fillings. If these were replaced with composite fillings, when I laughed everyone would see white teeth. After all the pros and cons were weighed (and being an indecisive Libran this took some time) I finally decided to go ahead.

Now this dentist was not keen to do this work on me because I told him I did not have injections during dental work. He tried very hard to convince me that there was a lot of work and the procedure would be painful. None of his arguments could sway me to have the injections. I am not scared of needles, which is just as well after all the intravenous chemotherapy and blood tests I needed, I just find I can channel the dental pain, with concentration, away from my mouth down my body and out through my toes. Sounds weird I will admit, it is just something I tried once many years ago and it worked so well I have done it since. The real benefit as I saw it was that immediately after the dental work I would feel fine and I would not dribble out of the side of my mouth.

Prior to the procedure we discussed the pros and cons of not having injections and he finally agreed to start work on a quarter of my mouth and if I wriggled or jumped he would use injections. The work was so intense he decided to do a quarter of my mouth at any one session, giving me time to recover. Also he could observe how the composite fillings reacted within my mouth between the appointments.

The first appointment arrived and I wriggled back into the dentist's chair and he lowered it into position. He fully explained what he was going to be doing. He put some hook type things around certain teeth and then fitted a rubber sheet (not the size of a bed sheet, my mouth is big, but not that big) on a few anchor teeth. Then he stretched the rubber taut across the top of my mouth by fixing it to the other hooked teeth. This was not pleasant. Then he fixed another rubber sheet across the bottom of my mouth in the same way. He seemed to manage to pop out the teeth he was going to be working on whilst still maintaining the taut rubber sheeting. I am guessing he popped out the teeth because I could not actually see what was happening, I could only feel it. The fitting of the rubber sheeting nearly caused me to ask for a morphine mask, let alone an injection.

Once he was fully satisfied that he had covered and sealed most of my mouth with rubber and he had access to the teeth he wanted to work on, he got started. Now most humans have around 32 teeth, give or take a couple of extractions, and I had about 10 teeth amalgam free. Working with these figures on this first appointment he drilled out the fillings from five of my teeth. Now I would like you to remember what it is like to have one filling before I go on. Now I want you to imagine, with full injections, having five replacement fillings (drilling out and re-filling) in one sitting (or should I be truthful and say within one lying down). Are you squirming yet?

Back to my appointment – he was a thorough dentist, determined not to leave any traces of amalgam wherever possible. It seemed to take a life time to complete the task. I lay there with my mouth stretched wide open feeling as taut as the rubber sheeting and wishing I had spent the dental money on a new carpet! Here is how I managed to go through the procedure without injections.

As soon as the drill started I closed my eyes and I mentally held my teeth in ready mode. Once the actual tooth had been selected and he was working on it I would use a pain wave system. I would create a pain wave which started in the mouth and rolled down my body. Thus, whenever I felt any pain, I would turn it into a pain wave. These waves would be rolling down my body and popping out of my toes. I thought it would be like creating waves as in a Cornish coast during a storm. Wrong! It was the equivalent of a tsunami. I was working as hard as the dentist, creating wave after wave. I had to fully concentrate and I had to work very quickly, creating waves, to keep on top of the pain. At the same time as creating the pain waves sweat was running down the back of my neck, over my back and down into the crack of my bottom. Sorry for all the details, only I want you to fully appreciate the situation I had found myself in. I had a pain tsunami in front and a slow moving sweat canal (not dental canal) down my back.

On a couple of occasions during this procedure, he accidently hit a nerve and my eyes would pop open in horror. Then I would mentally grab the pain and force it, in one move, not a rolling wave, just a fast rush of pain straight out of my toes. I liken this action to that of a rocket firework being let off and zooming out of my body, short cutting the journey from mouth to toes. This feat was very difficult to do and I only managed it because I was determined not to jump. The only indication the dentist could determine I was in pain, was by the fact that my eyes were closed most of the time and they popped open with a look of horror when sharp pain occurred.

Finally the ordeal was over; he was tired, I was exhausted and wet with sweat. Once he had removed all the rubber and bits of metal from my mouth he sat down and looked at me in surprise and said, 'When you told me no injections, I thought, that's what you say now, wait until the drill starts. Fair play to you, I am amazed you managed all those removals and fillings without injections. I would like to suggest we go for half your mouth next time, if you think you can stand it? All providing the composites settle down. The reason I suggest this is because you can handle the work and it takes a long time to secure the mouth before work can take place.'

'Well, it was tougher than I had anticipated but providing I can still opt for an injection if it gets too bad, I think I would like to get on with it,' I replied. I could reply without spitting at him because I could feel my tongue and teeth as I had not had any numbing injections.

It was agreed to do half a mouth next, and I had the rest of the removal of the amalgam and composite fitting in two more visits to the dentist. I left his surgery with my mouth full of resin composite fillings which felt a bit odd to start with but like anything in the mouth (now then, stop that smutty thought) you get used to it quite quickly.

I can honestly say that within days I felt better and within weeks I had extra energy and felt "younger." This is the only way I can describe it without gushing. Let me put in a caveat here; it could all be in my mind and be the result of autosuggestion, working overtime. I cannot say for sure what happened. All I know is that I felt better and I would do it all again regardless of the sheer pain and unimaginable discomfort suffered to remove the amalgam fillings.

You see, the final outcome, that of feeling more energised and healthier, far outweighs the scepticism and doomsayers. In the end it is not about them, it is about me taking those little steps, which on their own may or may not have an impact but when added together (compounding) they contributed to my well-being. That is what counts in my model of the world. If there is a remote chance that something was harming my body I would take action. If there was a remote chance that something might improve my health or well-being I would take action.

SUMMING UP

There is a lot of scientism around the mercury leakage from amalgam fillings and you will have to make your own mind up.

1   There is definitely mercury in amalgam fillings.

2   Mercury is definitely poisonous.

3   I spent many hours of research before embarking on amalgam removal.

4   I consider white fillings to look better than dark grey ones — in my model of the world.

CHAPTER SEVENTEEN

EARLY MENOPAUSE

All the stuff I did not know about menopause

Just to give you a bit of notice, I am about to cover a lot of detail on the topic of menopause. The main reason is because I feel that women and men may not typically know about or have heard about all the symptoms or about the many different remedies available. I took the opportunity to educate myself and I tried out quite a few of the possible remedies. I have covered them here.

Tamoxifen

From the first tablet I took of Tamoxifen (brand name: Nolvadex) my periods stopped. Now I cannot claim that it was the Tamoxifen which was the direct cause of the cessation of my periods, only that there seemed to be a correlation. I was not prepared for the menopause. I was not told (or if I was I certainly did not remember – hospital amnesia?) that there might be the possibility that I would be chemically forced through the menopause. I was 39 years young and to my mind the menopause was for women much older than me, surely?

The thing is, I started Tamoxifen as soon as I registered at the Royal Marsden Hospital before the surgery or the intravenous chemotherapy, which was a good thing because it turned out that my cancer was oestrogen (estrogen USA) receptor positive breast cancer and Tamoxifen is effective in preventing the recurrence of this. I was 39 years old.

At the time I was not in the least bit interested in any side effects of Tamoxifen or any of the drugs in the chemotherapy mixture. All I cared about was stopping the cancer and living. I am sure that if you told me I would have to do cartwheels (still cannot do them) every day for the rest of my life I would have volunteered to start immediately. It is terrifying being diagnosed with terminal cancer and I found I was willing to do whatever necessary to heal myself. Please do not judge me (unless you have also been terminally diagnosed); I was in shock.

At first it was quite nice not having to deal with the pre-menstrual tension (I had a lot of this, you can ask anyone who knew me), not having to cope with the blood loss and not having to buy the tampons (I was saving money). So without periods I was hassle free, what could be wrong with that?

Well, menopause changes the amount of oestrogen in your body and oestrogen keeps our skin soft and our bones hard, beside which, it also helps our female bodies to get ready for intimacy. There are many consequences to having less oestrogen in our bodies. In fact there is a list of them and it depends on your family history and your body, as to whether you will suffer from some or all of them.

Guess what? I do not know if it is family related or due to the chemically induced menopause but I suffered from each and every one of the side effects and I still suffer from some of them 23 years later. Hey, I would rather be bitching about my menopausal suffering than being dead, and when I put it in that context it is a no brainer. Anyway, I am happy to be alive and able to bitch, so stand back whilst I give it my best. I will take each consequence of menopause separately and explain how it affected me.

Flushes

I do not mean the toilet flush, I am talking about an altogether different flush. Hot flushes which, according to my cousin, are like electric power surges. She is so on the money with this description. You never know when it is going to happen so you cannot prepare; you do not know how long it will last; it is overwhelming; you have an urgent need to strip off all your clothes and dive into a cold sea and there is nothing you can do to stop the surges coming.

Years ago, in another life time, I used to see old women in twin-sets with fans and think that was old fashioned. The hot flushes changed this view. I used hand held and battery driven handbag size fans. I also dressed in layers so that when the power surges arrived I could take off the layers and then once the power surge had left my body, I would layer up again. When the power surge is over you rapidly lose body heat and become cold and sometimes clammy.

Night sweating

Night sweats are the same as hot flushes except they happen when you are asleep, which is really dreadful. You are awakened by a power surge of heat and sometimes you are drenched in sweat, soaking all the bed clothes. When you share a bed, it also affects your bed mate because your need to throw off the bedcovers is greater than your desire to be kind to your partner. Actually, you cannot think about anything except cooling down; it is an automatic reaction as you awaken, you have to grab the bed cover and get it off your body as soon as possible.

I have tried many different herbal remedies and cooling products. I once bought a water pillow, which worked really well as it kept my temperature even. You simply add cold water to the pillow and because it is filled with a type of natural absorbent material, it soaks up the water in a more even manner than water just sloshing around in a plastic bag. It was so good I decided I would take it on holiday to Spain.

When I arrived I asked my hosts if I could fill up my pillow, and I added about four pints of cold water. They looked a little alarmed and I reassured them by telling them I had used the pillow for many months without any problems. I think I did not put the stopper fully into the pillow. All I can remember is waking up in the middle of a dream, where I was swimming in the sea off the beautiful Saunton Sands beach, thinking to myself, "I still feel wet from the swim" only to realise the bed was soaked with nearly four pints of water! I had bought one for my mother as a gift and she loved it until hers did the same. We have both given up on the idea.

Fans

Going back to fans, Pete was fed up with being woken with me trying to cool down during the night, so one day he came back to our three bedroom house in Bournemouth with two massive industrial ceiling fans. The fans had three speeds and when he had fixed them into the two main bedrooms he proudly called me upstairs for a demonstration. The slowest speed was very fast and very cooling – I was impressed and expressed my delight.

'Just you wait,' he said as he clicked the fan to speed two which was so powerful it ruffled the bedding.

'Wow, that is strong!' I carefully mentioned.

Then with a pleased flick of his wrist he reached the top speed of the fan. Well it was so powerful it was hard to stand below it and it sounded as if it had the power to take off the roof. You could not speak for the noise and the wind tunnel effect.

'That should sort out your night sweats,' he smugly announced once the fan had slowly ground to a halt and we could draw breath.

'It is wonderful,' I said, as I was very pleased with this turn of events. I think we both knew this demonstration was going to be the last time the top speed would be used.

Many years later we moved into our new spectacular home (designed by Pete) and he insisted the builder add to each of the main bedrooms a remote controlled electric ceiling fan. The fans fitted by the builder are also for use in offices and factories but they are nowhere near as powerful as the ones we left in Bournemouth. I still suffer from night sweats at least four or five times a week so I am truly grateful for the remote fan which never needs dusting because it is used summer and winter.

Vaginal dryness

Vaginal dryness is not discussed by anyone until you suffer from it. The menopause is the normal cessation of the female menstrual cycle. Vaginal dryness is an effect of menopause, which in turn might cause sexual dysfunction due to the pain caused by friction owing to lack of vaginal fluid. I mentioned this dryness and pain to the oncologist at one of my hospital visits. She sympathised and asked me if I had tried any remedies.

'Yes, I have tried the normal sexual lubricants available over the counter but nothing seems to work for me.'

She looked at her notes and 'Umm, ah. Okay, well you know that your cancer was oestrogen receptor positive?'

'Yes,' I said.

'Normally we would recommend HRT (hormone replacement therapy) but in your case we could not be sure of the effects this might have on your cancer. We could try oestrogen suppositories or creams and again I need to stress that with your cancer being oestrogen receptor positive, it is not something I would recommend. I suggest you take some time to think about this and chat about it with your partner,' she said.

I agreed to chat to Pete about this option and we both agreed the risk was too great. So at my next appointment with the oncologist I told her we did not want to go down this route.

'Well, this means that the normal treatments we would recommend will not be available to you,' she lamented and she suggested I look at alternative options of vaginal lubrication.

Vitamin E

So I looked at supplements and found that vitamin E supplements had good reviews on the reduction of the symptoms of hot flashes and vaginal dryness because it boosts the female sex hormone oestrogen. There, in the last word, was the reason I have not tried this option. The risk was too great for me to consider taking vitamin E supplements. I therefore decided to change my diet and include foods high in vitamin E, such as Brazil nuts, spinach, broccoli, peanut butter, almonds, kiwi and mango. There are some seeds like flax and sunflower but although I tried them I kept forgetting to sprinkle them on my food.

My reasoning for the diet additions was that unlike supplements which tend to give higher doses, natural food high in vitamin E would be processed in a more natural slower manner, and in my model of the world, would mean less risk. I do not know if this is scientifically true, but it is what I decided to do. I did not notice any vast improvement in my vaginal dryness, however I did notice that my skin and nails improved.

Evening primrose oil

I also took evening primrose oil (Oenothera biennis) tablets for a while. As I did not notice a change in the frequency or power of the flushes (day or night) I eventually stopped. There are some pretty hairy reported side effects with the blood and the immune system which did not inspire me. It has also been stated that if you are taking any anticoagulants or phenothiazines (psychotherapeutic organic compound) you should avoid taking evening primrose oil. All of this information put me off continuing taking it.

Herbal remedies

I tried some of the herbal remedies. I took Black Cohosh (Actaea racemosa, Cimicifuga racemosa) for a short period as there was some scientific awareness for possibly reducing hot flushes but there was some confusion on whether it worked like oestrogen and as you are aware, I was not prepared to take any risks with products containing oestrogen. Also, there was some negative linking to liver problems and I felt I would not go down this route because of the risks, albeit small risks. It was not for me, the risks outweighed the gains. I stopped taking the tablets so I cannot comment on its efficacy.

I liked the thought of taking a traditional Chinese medicine and Dong Quai (Angelica sinensis) has been used by the Chinese for gynaecological conditions for over 1,000 years. I did not find any reduction in the hot flushes and gave up. It is said that Dong Quai should not be used if you are taking blood clotting medication, or if you have fibroids because complications can arise. I decided not to take the risk.

I took Ginseng (Panax ginseng or Panax quinquefolius) for quite some time (about two years) as it seemed to help me with the mood swings and general feeling of well-being. It did nothing to alleviate the hot flushes.

On one of the visits to the Royal Marsden Hospital I bumped into one of the nurses who worked on the Ellis Ward whilst I was in and out of it with greater frequency than was normal, hence she remembered me. We got chatting and I mentioned the problems I was having with the menopause and the fact I could not have HRT because of my oestrogen receptor positive cancer. She suggested I look into natural progesterone creams as she had heard that they could reduce hot flushes. At the time it was difficult to buy natural progesterone cream. I found one source and bought one tube, only when I went back to buy some more, I was told they no longer sold it, something to do with government intervention.

I eventually sourced it out of Guernsey and used it for over a year. It did reduce the severity of my hot flushes, only not sufficiently enough for me to continue using the cream when the difficulty of sourcing was factored into the decision.

Acupuncture

I also tried acupuncture as I had heard that some women found relief from their menopausal symptoms by visiting an acupuncturist. Some doctors agree acupuncture is a satisfactory alternative to HRT especially where women are suffering from depression and hot flushes. Again, there are cynics who say any acupuncture benefits are purely the result of the placebo effect. My argument, as you well know by now, is that if there are any benefits then my outcome is being reached. I really don't care if this is because it can be scientifically proven or is just the placebo effect. An interesting point is that some health insurance plans cover acupuncture, among other alternative treatments, which seems to concur that it works.

I was referred to the acupuncturist by a delegate on one of the courses I was running. We had lunch together and I had one of my power surges and I started to de-robe whilst searching for my fan, when she mentioned that she visited an acupuncturist who had helped her get her flushes under control. I left with the contact details and quickly made my appointment. I am not scared of needles and I have a high pain threshold, only I was uncomfortable with the procedure. I was surprised that the needles were long and that they were not just placed into position, she wriggled them around every now and then. I probably did not help matters as I kept getting tense. I came out of the acupuncturist's clinic knowing I would not be returning.

When I look back on the things I tried, nothing much worked for me. However, in some instances like acupuncture, perhaps I should have given it more time. I think some of the reasons behind my not getting the results other women achieved from some of the alternative therapies could be due to the fact that I was suffering from a chemically induced menopause at a relatively young age. I am not sure.

Bone thinning

Thinning of the bones (osteopenia) is also associated with the menopause and the Royal Free Hospital was keeping a very close eye on my bones because of the trial drug programme I was on. This meant I had MRI (magnetic resonance imaging) scans. One time I was given an injection of dye into a vein in my left arm, another time I was given a drink beforehand. Both were to introduce into my body a contrast medium. This contrast medium can help the images from the scan to show up more clearly.

I think I am a bit odd, in the fact that I did not mind the scans one little bit even though you are shoved in a long tube for around 30 minutes. I am not claustrophobic as I found out during the helicopter journey I mentioned in chapter 5 *Setbacks*. The machine is very noisy, but I was given headphones so that the person operating the scanner could give me information during the scan. I used to treat the event like an excuse to lie down and being highly auditory, as previously mentioned in chapter 14 *Light And Laughter*, meant I could play songs in my head. I was always a little sad when the operator would say, 'That's it. We are done now and we will be bringing you out' or words to that effect.

I have read that weight bearing exercise helps reduce bone loss and can increase bone density. Here is a good webpage to give you some ideas on what you can do if you are worried about bone loss: *http://www.webmd.com/osteoporosis/living-with-osteoporosis-7/exercise-weight-bearing*. There are seven different weight bearing activities and what is said here about Tai Chi is amazing and I quote: *"A study reported in Physician and Sportsmedicine found that tai chi could slow bone loss in postmenopausal women. The women, who did 45 minutes of tai chi a day, five days a week for a year, enjoyed a rate of bone loss up to three-and-a-half times slower than the non-tai-chi group."*

I did go to Tai Chi classes one winter and found it really interesting. I have decided to start again now that I have read these amazing results and once I have finished this book I will look for a local class.

Mood swings

One of the well-known symptoms of menopause is mood swings and I yo-yoed across the human mood spectrums (I did not know this existed until the moment I looked on the internet and there it was – human mood spectrum!). My mood swings were erratic, and uncontrollable. I could find myself in floods of tears, flushed with happiness or so angry I would find myself shouting for no reason.

Weight gain

Weight gain is also a symptom of the menopause, but as I had already gained loads of weight during the chemotherapy, I could not honestly say if it was because of chemotherapy, menopause or just me pigging out during bouts of self-pity.

Dry skin and hair

Dry hair and skin has always been a problem for me and this was exacerbated by the menopause. I used many different hair and skin products but there are none that stand out for me to recommend to you, excluding vitamin E. You can take it as a supplement (read the contraindications) or you can eat the foods I have previously mentioned which are high in vitamin E.

Rosacea

Rosacea, what is this I hear you say? I was introduced to the word as Acne Rosacea which when both words are put together make more sense to me. During menopause, women can sometimes get red pimples and bumps appearing and it is easy to assume they have acne. Actually the skin changes are related to a condition known as rosacea. I noticed that the whole of my nose and some surrounding areas started to become red. Then a patch of red skin appeared in between my eye brows and one covered my entire chin. It was not a pretty sight and I learned that redness is also a symptom of rosacea. Even after reading many studies on the subject, there does not seem to be any specific causative factor, just a lot of different things which can cause it. Rosacea is not solely as a result of the menopause. I only learnt about it because I developed it during my menopause. It is said that if you already have rosacea before your menopause the hot flushes from the menopause can exacerbate your rosacea.

Rosacea can present itself as red patches (this is what I had) or you can have persistent red spots. Some women get thread-like skin capillaries (telengiectasia) which show up on the surface of the face and some people are affected by their eyelids becoming swollen or reddened (blepharitis). I am lucky in that I only suffer from the red patches and for the most part if I am careful they are not so bad. Actually, I had a very bad cycle accident in 2010 where I scraped my face along a tarmac road, thus, experiencing my second trip in an air ambulance. So the rosacea which seemed quite important before the accident has slipped into the shadows of my facial scarring. Every cloud has a silver lining.

The National Rosacea Society has a good website which might help you as it gives some useful ideas on how to reduce the symptoms. They have a newsletter and lots of pictures which might help you identify if rosacea is what you are suffering from. The first thing I would suggest is to keep a food and drinks diary to see if there is a correlation with the rosacea flare-up and what you are putting into your body. Then stop or reduce any foodstuffs or drink which you know exacerbates the rosacea. I found that if I ate any foods containing chilli this would cause a flare-up. I always wear a sunscreen now and most foundation make-up these days contains sunscreens within their ingredients. I also avoid any skincare products which seem to aggravate it. I recommend you visit a dermatologist as he or she will be able to advise you on the best things to do for your condition.

Every woman is different and will experience the menopause symptoms to a greater or a lesser extent. One of my close friends, Prue van der Nat, sailed through the menopause with only a couple of hot flushes and a few night sweats. Actually, I am so envious I could strike her off my friend list, only I would miss her dreadfully and I love her to bits. She taught me how to wear scarves in the early days of my cancer treatment, what is not to love?

I suffered quite severely from hot flushes for over 15 years and I still have regular night sweats. I think the night sweats are a family thing; my mother is still having night sweats and she is 89 years young. So I do not hold out much hope of reducing them in the near future, especially as I seem to have exhausted most of the medical and alternative remedies.

Sometime later, I had to go back to the same oncologist I had spoken to about the vaginal dryness because a cervical cancer test I was given showed some irregularities. It turned out that I had stage 3 pre-cancer cells present. They removed the cells by cryotherapy which destroys abnormal tissue on the cervix by freezing it. It sounds grim, but it was not – liquid carbon dioxide (CO_2) was placed next to the abnormal tissue via a probe for five minutes. I was warned that I could feel a sensation of cold and/or a sensation of warmth which could spread to the upper body and face. I had both. It was weird the sensation of warmth; I was used to hot flushes but this was different as it was a slower burn. It was all over quickly and on my return visit I was given the all clear.

SUMMING UP

Menopause has many symptoms, and I had most of them for which I explored lots of different remedies.

1. I had hot flushes like power surges and night sweats that made the bed wet.

2. I suffered vaginal dryness and tried lots of different things.

3. I was concerned about my bones thinning so I learnt Tai chi.

4. Mood swings and weight gain were part of the experience.

5. My hair became very dry as did my skin and I also suffered with rosacea. Vitamin E worked for me.

6. I was diagnosed with vaginal cancer and had cryotherapy.

CHAPTER EIGHTEEN

PICTURE OF HEALTH

Visualisation, affirmation mantras and movement

Prior to developing cancer I was quite bigoted and narrow minded and I would have considered personal development and all of its weird and wacky methodology just that – weird and wacky. I was judgemental and I believed that my model of the world was the only valid model of the world. I probably would not have considered life coaching as a career choice (although at that time it did not exist) as I would not have understood what it was about. Nor would I have been prepared to investigate something which suggested in its title that my life needed fixing. I most definitely would not have attended any Mind & Body events (even if they had been around to attend at the time, which they weren't) let alone been a speaker at one. Yes, I have now been a speaker at Mind & Body events, NLP conferences and coaching conferences, all of which would not have happened if I had not survived cancer.

One of the many things I have learnt along the way is to put my trust into some of the wacky ideas or methods of self-development and go for it. It has been this trust which has opened the door of discovery into a whole new world. A world where the mind matters and thoughts affect everything. What is truly great about this revelation is the freedom to take control of my body and mind. One of the important things I have learnt is to keep going even when you think no changes are taking place. With some of the activities I could easily have given up before I reached the first hurdle, let alone at the first hurdle.

Law of Attraction

For me the strangest is the Law of Attraction. There are many varieties of how this works and what works best. The basic premise is that if you think about what you want, if you picture it clearly, if you tell yourself concisely what you want and if you feel like you already have it, then the Law of Attraction will work to bring it to you. The challenge is to keep out the negative thoughts about anything or anybody. After four decades of negative thought patterns I found the idea a bit preposterous let alone actually taking any actions. With an attitude like that I would seem doomed to fail and it is amazing that I did not fail.

Eventually, I decided I would give it a go. I thought about all the things I wanted and wrote them down. Even as I was writing what I wanted I could hear my inner voice saying, 'This won't work.' The Law of Attraction swings into action for both positive and negative requests. So I was proved to be right, it did not work! What I love about the Law of Attraction is that it cannot be wrong because if it works then you get what you want and you are happy. If it fails, it fails because you allowed it to fail by your negative thoughts, a brilliant business strategy.

Honestly, the physical requests have worked really well for me but the material requests have been a little off the mark. This could be explained by the fact that I am fully focused on my health and only partially focused on my wealth. Therefore, the wealth side of things did not bring the same results because I was not putting in the work and energy needed to make it happen. I will share with you the process I used (which is not correct in the pure sense of Law of Attraction methods) concerning my health. I used a combination of Law of Attraction, visualisation, affirmations, incantations and physiology.

I will take each part individually so you can understand how the whole works, starting with knowing what you want. This sound ridiculous, why wouldn't you know what you want? Well, if you have never before considered exactly (I mean precisely in great detail) what you want besides perhaps the obvious such as a mansion house and flashy car, expensive jewellery and any other unspecific thing, this will come as a great surprise. Taking the time to sit down in front of a screen or piece of paper and actually describe in great detail the item you want is much harder than just saying a mansion house or good health.

When I started this process I said I wanted to be in good health. So, what did good health mean to me? You see good health can just mean that I am alive, or I can run a marathon (highly unlikely, not because I could not do it but because I do not want to do it), it could mean I weigh a certain weight. Being specific is all important. I started with good health and then I began to describe what this meant in more specific terms.

I wanted to be fit – still too general. I amended this to being fit enough to complete a 5k race. Then I made it even more specific, being fit enough to either jog or walk from start to finish in a Cancer Research 5k race for life. Then I thought about it a bit more and realised that I did not just want to complete the race, I needed to be fit enough to complete the 5k race for life and I did not want to suffer aches, pain or stiffness afterwards. Now I was in trouble, because you cannot use negatives in your Law of Attraction wants list. This bit I always found difficult because, as I have previously mentioned, I was negatively wired. My natural inclination in those days was to think negatively first. The wonderful thing is being able to recognise the negative pattern and then taking action to change it.

So the first step for me was to spot the negative thought and then I needed to work on turning a negative statement into a positive statement. The positive statement needs to give a positive outcome, for example, let's take the words "not suffering" which seems good to me, who would want to suffer? If you look at "not suffering" you will realise that there are two negatives, the word "not" and the word "suffering", so I had to turn this around.

'I want to be fit enough to complete the 5k race for life and walk easily with gladness afterwards.'

This worked; I completed the race and I could walk afterwards, I did not suffer from stiffness or pain in the following days. This could have also been the result of lots of practise beforehand, I will never know for definite.

Then I thought about the cancer and what I wanted with this. Again I could not use the word cancer because it is a negative word so stating that I was cancer free would not work. What exactly did I want? I was a bit stumped about the answer to that question.

Incantation

In the 1920s a Frenchman called Émil Coué introduced a mantra "Every day, and in every way, I am becoming better and better." I cannot remember how I first heard of this saying/mantra but I thought it sounded like a good idea and something easy to concentrate on. I have adjusted it to suit my model of the world and a phraseology I am more comfortable with.

I get healthier every day, I get healthier in every way.

This worked for me and it is easy to adapt.

I get (blank) every day and I get (blank) in every way. The word in brackets can represent anything you like: healthier, happier, thinner, wealthier, wiser, you think of it, you put it in the brackets.

Once I started chanting this I realised that it can be easily broken down to fit the American Armed Forces jogging chant which I mention in Chapter 13 Race for my Life

'Dah duh, dah duh, dah dah dah = I get, healthier, ev ery day

Dah duh, dah duh, dah dah dah' = I get, healthier, in ev ery way

So now I have an incantation (mantra or chant) which can be an "I CAN tation". This representation of the word is not of my originality, I remember seeing it somewhere either on a website, in a blog or book, and thinking that is great. I can use this incantation easily when I jog, walk or simply think about it. I often use it when I find myself thinking negatively about something or someone; saying this chant distracts me from the negativity and allows me to refocus.

One of my favourite mantras is 'I am happy, healthy, wealthy, wise, healed and whole' which is also easy to say, but sadly I have not been able to fit it into the American Armed Forces jogging chant. I use this mantra every day. In Chapter 5 Setbacks, I mention that when I shower I also complete a manual lymphatic drainage routine on my special arm (the one with only a few lymph nodes). At the same time I am massaging my arm, I tell my arm, 'I love you' and I also say my mantra 'I am happy, healthy, wealthy, wise, healed and whole.' Now, if you think this is wacky, I suggest you prepare yourself as I also give my arm a kiss after I have said 'I love you.' I will admit, the first time I kissed my arm I felt really odd and even though I was in the shower alone, I still looked around to see if anyone was watching me. I felt like a real fool. It took many times and many kisses later before I felt comfortable with this. Now it is all part of my daily routine and it is a great way to start the day.

Here is another tip, on talking to yourself. When I am alone in a bathroom and there is a mirror, I look into my eyes and say 'I love you.' This was also weird and strange at first. With practise I now do this with ease. Again I cannot remember if I read this or was told this, as it was a long time ago. I do know it works. My body, the only one I will ever have, knows with complete certainty that I love it and respect it. Remember back in Chapter 13 Race for my Life I mentioned a guy called Doctor Emoto Masaru who believed that water could react to both positive and negative thoughts and words. Well our bodies are made up of mostly water (around 50-70%) and if there is a remote chance that saying nice things to water works, I am happy to tell my 50-70% that I love it and, hopefully, my body performs for me and keeps itself healthy. Have some fun, look in the mirror and into your own eyes and tell yourself 'I love you' and see how you feel about that. I bet you will smile back at yourself.

Visualisation

I touched on visualisation during Chapter 11 Cancer of Thoughts and Chapter 10 Know your Enemy. In a nut-shell, after you have clearly defined what you want, you then visualise yourself as already having achieved or acquired the thing you clearly defined.

In the film, The Secret, based on a story by Rhonda Byrne, one of the cast of presenters, John Assaraf, talks about the power of having a vision board which is a pictorial representation of goals. To create your own board, find a pin board or you can create an electronic version possibly on Pinterest or a similar site. Once you have your board, you select photos and symbols of your wants/goals and you pin them to your board, which you look at frequently. I have my board as the background on my computer, which I look at every day when I log on and log off. Every day look at your vision board to remind your unconscious, inner conscious mind, or subconscious what it is exactly that you want.

A very effective visualisation method I have used successfully for many years, is to make a movie with you as the star achieving the goal or getting what you want. The key thing to concentrate on is that you are the leading star and you need to be alive in your movie. This is not a movie you just watch, it should be a performance you take part in.

is is an action movie, in full colour, with all the sounds
would be hearing when you achieve your goal. Who
be in your movie and what will they be doing or saying
ou? Think about how you will be feeling. Will there
be any smells (it is good to add in smells) and think about
what tastes are in your mouth? Involve all your five senses
and make the experience real so your body as well as your
mind, is convinced it has already happened. Have some fun
when making your movie. When you replay your movie,
because you are having fun you will release endorphins into
your system and endorphins equal a feel good factor. Get
physically involved, which means that you need to change
your body posture when creating your movie and put your
body into the same position when playing back the movie
as this speeds up the process.

I have a body position when I am sad or about to cry
and a completely different body pose when I am happy and
ecstatic. Get to know your body and the poses you put your
body into because you can affect the way you feel simply
by changing your body position. For example, it is hard to
cry when you hold your head up, with your chin high and
a smile on your face. Body positions are normally executed
on an unconscious level and I am saying be conscious of your
body. You can consciously choose your body position and by
doing so, you can bring more happiness into your life. This
is especially important if you are feeling sad or low. Simply
change your sad body pose into your happy one and if possible dance! Actions like dancing will rapidly and completely
change how you feel. You can choose how you feel and you
can select your body pose to support your feelings. Make
better choices.

My movies have altered over the years depending on what I want to achieve health wise. If I have entered into a charity run or more recently a charity daffodil walk of 10k, I create a movie of me happily and healthily striding along with my friends, admiring the views. I am chanting 'I am happy, healthy, wealthy, wise, healed and whole,' which is one of my favourite incantations. The movie's endings are always with my arms up (in the movie and whilst remembering the movie) pushing my chest out as I cross over the finish line with a big smile on my face. I glance over to my friends and they are also smiling. I feel triumphant, joyous, happy and healthy. I have a slight sweet taste in my mouth and I can smell freshly cut grass.

Think very carefully what you want to achieve, write it down in specific detail. Create a mantra and an action movie and play it often.

SUMMING UP

The Law of Attraction is a powerful methodology, once you know what you want.

1   The mind matters and thoughts affect everything.

2   The Law of Attraction needs specifics to work.

3   Visualisation is a colourful experience.

4   Mantras, I CAN tations.

5   Movement makes the movie more realistic, more powerful, more memorable and can have more impact.

CHAPTER NINETEEN

FROM CANCER TO COACHING

Every cloud has a silver lining

When I was diagnosed with cancer over 23 years ago I was told I would be dead within nine months of the diagnosis. I had an aggressive form of breast cancer which had spread into my lymphatic system. I was not making plans! There is a Jewish saying: "Man plans, God laughs."

As you will have read in the earlier chapters, I organised a farewell birthday party thinking it would be my last. I have had many, many more since then. You will remember that I could not keep a job offer more than a couple of days because as soon as the employer found out that I had had cancer I was "persona non grata." I was lucky when my freelance computer trainer application found its way into the hands of a very desperate lady who gave me a laptop and a job.

I absolutely loved the job as a freelance computer trainer – I had learnt to be a computer trainer way back in the 1980s when I worked for Wang Laboratories Inc. I was merrily working for the company in Bournemouth as a freelance trainer and most of the training was done at the headquarters of a large international bank. Then the government brought in some new rules which roughly stated, that if a freelancer works for only one company even if the freelancer is placed by that company into many different companies, the freelancer is deemed to be an employee of the agent company. Wow, this put the cat amongst the pigeons.

This move by the government encouraged me to look around for other computer training companies to freelance for. The plus side of the government's actions was that every freelancer had to find another company to work for and all the training companies encouraged this as they did not want to become the employer. I looked through my old address book and I contacted a lady who worked as a contractor for me back in the Wang days. She had successfully set up her own computer company working out of beautiful Malmesbury and I became one of her freelance trainers. I now had two suppliers and a wide variety of work and workplaces. Around that time, I heard through the grapevine one of the trainers who worked for me in the Wang days was now the training manager for a large computer training company based in Wimbledon. I gave him a call and started to work for him on a freelance basis.

The delegates on the courses I delivered for the Wimbledon training company were giving me excellent reviews on my training and knowledge. I was asked if I would be happy to train myself on their range of management skills programmes. I was delighted because they had very high standard management courses. So, as well as being paid to deliver the computer training, I started to sit-in on their management course portfolio. I really enjoyed the range of courses and because I had already held many management roles in the past, I used my experience and knowledge to elaborate the training points.

They had within their portfolio a one week management course and it was one of the most outstanding courses I have had the privilege to co-deliver. The course had been written for them by some business guru and was very cleverly constructed. It was a hugely complicated role play set around a coast guard station, with a variety of difficult situations thrown in. The delegates eventually get themselves into a muddle, forgetting critical things and blaming each other.

On the final day of the course the whole group (led by one of the delegate trainee managers) would have to run a coast guard station, which another of the delegates (two days previous) had been tasked with setting up, not knowing at the time, the station would be used later in the week. The delegate had been creating job roles, putting up the maps, identifying tasks that needed to be performed etc...

Also on this last day, two trainers would be working in an adjoining room with walkie-talkie and phone contact with the coast guard station. Reading a script, each trainer would take separate roles, one on the walkie-talkie and the other on the phone. The trainers would start gently notifying the coast guard that boats were leaving port; they would ask if it was safe to go out windsurfing; one would ring up asking about weather reports. Then out of nowhere, the Met Office (a trainer) announced a weather warning and mayhem would always ensue. The trainers would now be working the phones and walkie-talkie at the same time announcing people in trouble, boats calling in Pan Pan (just below Mayday) and other large ships asking if they can dock. A doddery old man (trainer) rang up blocking the phone line for a long time.

As you can imagine the delegates get into a real mess, forget to do critical things and eventually start blaming each other (which is exactly how the course was designed). At that point one of the trainers would announce that the boat which was in serious trouble, the one who called in a Pan Pan, had now moved up to a full Mayday. The other trainer simultaneously announcing that the rescue team sent (by the delegates) to the windsurfers had arrived too late and there had been a fatality. This news always stops the coast guard station in its tracks until someone remembers there is still a Mayday to deal with.

Eventually the exercise is wound up and after lunch the review of the interactions takes place. It is the fastest learning of bad management skills they will ever endure and they all learn the importance of the true role of a manager and the poisonous effects of a blame culture. I loved this course because of the massive growth in skills and competencies the delegates attained.

I was also asked around that time, if I would consider delivering the one day company introduction course for a bank in Bournemouth and although I did not have a clue (what is new there?) I agreed to give it a go. The course ran every Monday morning (they recruited a lot of people in those days) and I turned up to observe. It was fascinating as it covered the normal introduction course information, such as employee handbook, restaurant facilities, etc., and it also included money laundering (not how to launder money), what money laundering is, how it works and how to spot it during normal business transactions. I delivered this course for well over a year and really enjoyed it.

The interesting thing is, when you are a freelance trainer you do not get paid for learning new courses, no matter how long it takes or the number of days you are required to sit-in and observe. Also, not only do you not get paid for the sit-ins, you are losing money because you are not working. This means there is not a high take up of freelancers willing to learn new courses, which worked in my favour as I love to learn new courses. My investment paid huge dividends as I had a much larger skill set and there was always work for me if I wanted it.

Two of the courses I delivered were coaching courses – to train employees and managers how to coach. For the managers, their course involved how to coach team members to achieve greater performance levels, how to coach team members to take greater responsibility and coaching within the appraisal system. For the employees the coaching was related to task training, where a member of staff who was competent in one task had to train another member of staff in that task by using coaching.

Sometime later, I was introduced to a business man who wanted a professional coach trainer to write a life coaching course and he asked me if I would write the course materials and run the course as the course director. I agreed to do the work but only on a freelance basis and I ran his course for about a year. I became very unhappy with the numbers of people being pushed through the course and we had many irreconcilable ethical differences. It was a battle I was not prepared to enter into. I also took into consideration, because of the research I had undertaken, that stress is a known contributor to cancer and I consistently avoid any stressful situations.

Having parted company with him, I decided to set up my own life coach training company and at the same time I spent the year writing *The Life Coaching Handbook, Everything you need to be an effective life coach*, published by Crown House Publishing. I did not know at the time of writing the book or at publication (a year later), that my book was the first book in the world to be written on how to become a life coach. There were several books on life coaching including Fiona Harrold's *Be Your Own Life Coach: How to Take Control of Your Life and Achieve Your Wildest Dreams* but not one book on how to actually become a life coach and run your own business practice.

I launched my book and my life coaching business. I found that the really good thing about running my own business was that I was in control of the standard of training and I could set a limit on the number of delegates within a course. Having previously not being allowed to make changes to the course because it was not my business, I now had complete freedom to create a full diploma course. I included the latest enhanced learning techniques; I produced a multi-media experience and designed a copyright values elicitation form. I created a completely different coaching course which enhanced and accelerated learning whilst constructing an environment for complete coaching immersion.

I continuously enhance, modify and update the course materials as new ideas and methodologies come along, which keeps my interest and enthusiasm for the course high. The original course had to be completed within six months as I thought this would keep the delegates motivated and I would have a marking schedule with everything clearly defined. When I researched the training courses in the USA from whence life coaching came, a six month course seemed to be the standard practice.

One of my first delegates rang me about four months into his course in a terrible state. He told me that his son was a drug addict and had completely ransacked his home, stealing anything he could sell and smashing everything else. He was worried about not completing the course on time. I reassured him that I would extend the course completion date for him and I would mark his work when he was ready to hand it in. This got me thinking about the deadline and how it would affect people and I decided against all "normal" coach training practice to make my course deadline free of restrictions. Delegates could complete the course within a time frame to suit themselves. Eventually, most of the other coach training courses have followed suit.

I worked hard to attain external verification of high standards and my course now has the top accreditation from the International Institute of Coaching and Mentoring (IIC&M). When the course was running successfully I decided I would write another book. This time I would share the majority of the learning from the business courses I used to run and from my own business experiences. This was a fascinating journey for me and *The Business Coaching Handbook: Everything you need to be your own Business Coach,* was written. Here is what one of my business clients wrote about the book.

'Curly's clarity of thinking coupled with her ability to apply personal development concepts to real world situations has proved invaluable in both my personal and business life. I would have no hesitation in recommending her work to any aspiring entrepreneur looking to leverage some quality ideas in their business.'

—NIGEL WINSHIP, MANAGING DIRECTOR.

A year later I had written and published *The Personal Success Handbook: Everything you need to be Successful,* which completed the Handbook Series. In this book I wanted to redefine the accepted view of success and give the reader the option to decide what success actually means for them. Prior to my cancer diagnosis, I was preoccupied with equating my success with accumulating money, collecting chattels and being seen in the best places. I had never stopped to think about the treadmill I had created for myself, nor had I taken the time to decide what success actually meant to me. The first chapter is all about deciding what success means to an individual regardless of the accepted norm.

There are chapters on health, emotional control, dealing with relationships in a positive and constructive manner, changing limiting beliefs (although I do not cover the intervention Museum of Old Beliefs from chapter 15) and altering our personal rule books. I do include a wealth generation section which shows you how to determine your net worth and how to generate further income if you need it. This is supported by chapters on how to get a job and be successful within your career. Here is what one of my business friends wrote about the book.

'I love books that make a difference — and the Personal Success Handbook is one of those! Packed full of useful ideas, it gives direction and a sense of purpose as you read it. It focuses attention on the practical and possible action steps needed to move anyone's life forward in all areas. The illustrative stories add to our understanding and the many exercises and activities woven throughout the text, encourage us gently but firmly, along the path of change. Easy to read, free of jargon, thought provoking and purposeful — a book for those people serious about life improvement — so LET'S DO IT!'

—GILL FIELDING.
(A Secret Millionaire, ITV Channel 4)

The interesting thing about the cancer is that if it had not happened I would never have considered coaching as a career and more importantly, I would not have become an international bestselling author. How cool is that? I absolutely adore my profession and it is most definitely my purpose in this lifetime. I consider myself to be very lucky to earn a living growing and developing others. I have had the honour and privilege of working with some amazingly talented and original people, which is the most rewarding and fun thing I have ever done. Without the cancer diagnosis this would not have happened. I have a lot to be grateful for.

SUMMING UP

I believe that setbacks are the universe showing you that you are going the wrong way. It is a nudge towards your true vocation.

1   Being forced to change direction was a wonderful thing for me.

2   I became flexible and brave.

3   Sometimes I earnt more money by firstly earning less.

4   I recognise stressful situations and do all in my power to avoid them.

CHAPTER TWENTY

DAILY DOZEN

Things I do

There are certain things that I do on a regular basis and although I have shared most of them with you throughout the book, I wanted to put the things which I think are important in the maintenance of my health in one chapter so you can easily find them. If you have started this book at this chapter I just want you to be aware that the daily dozen is not the whole picture of how I dealt with the death diagnosis. It is only the 12 things I do now on a regular basis, 23 years later. The order of the daily dozen is not significant for me; I just do them in no particular order of importance, every day or once a week.

Daily Dozen

1   **Walking** – every day I make sure I have done some form of exercise. During the week I walk about four to five miles a day around the country lanes. I power walk for

the most part, excluding the hills where I generally slow down and take my time. When I say power walk, I think that is a bit of an exaggeration to be truthful because for some people a power walk is just below the speed of jogging and it causes breathlessness and sweating. I walk fast but not so fast that I am out of breath or break out in a sweat. I walk to maintain my health, not for any competitive reasons.

Monday to Friday I sit at a desk, sometimes for eight to ten hours, looking at a computer. I do get up every hour or less to grab a drink or visit the toilet to get rid of said drink. I know all this sitting is not good for my body, so come rain (and it does a lot of that in the West Country) or shine, I go for my walk.

2   **Vitamins and minerals** – I supplement my diet with vitamins. I know there are scientific studies which say that if you eat a balanced diet you do not need them. The challenge is that I cannot be sure the food I eat has been grown in soil which has all the nutrients I need. There is a strong possibility my balanced diet will be lacking in something. So I take a multi vitamin/mineral supplement every day to act as a back-up to the food I eat.

At the same time I take a 1000 milligram tablet of Vitamin C (ascorbic acid). Vitamin C is a water soluble vitamin which the body does not store and cannot make. I have to consume it. It is essential for healing wounds, it is also an antioxidant, supporting my immune system, and it forms part of the absorption of iron facilitation within my body.

I also take selenium because, like Vitamin C, it is essential for my body and my body does not make it. There is a lot of scepticism about the benefits of taking selenium. However, the information I read stated that there was not sufficient selenium in soil these days and being a non-meat eater I would have less in my food. So I take tablets to supplement.

I take various other supplements depending on the changes in my state of health.

3   **I CAN tations** – Every day I chant (another word for incantation). One of my favourite ones is, 'I am happy, healthy, wealthy, wise, healed and whole' which I say in a rhythmic voice as I walk. Usually, I chant this mantra after I have completed my gratitude statements.

4   **Fruit** – Before the diagnosis I would say I was a fruit eater, which was true, only I did not eat very much fruit nor did I eat fruit on a regular basis. I liked fruit and I would eat it in a fruit salad, in a pie, if it was the dessert on offer such as strawberries and cream. I would not eat it regularly as a fruit on its own and when I look back, I realise now that if I was given the choice, I would never choose a fruit instead of a flapjack, scone or muffin. I would never buy fruit if there was a chocolate bar instead. So although I ate fruit, I was not a fruit eater.

Now, I eat a variety of fruits every day and cannot imagine a day without it. In the summer I eat a mixed fruit salad for breakfast and in the winter I eat blueberries on my porridge. I would make smoothies or fruit juices, only it's too much like hard work and I cannot be bothered.

I am a busy lady, so I eat fruit whole. I did buy a big juicing machine shortly after diagnosis, which sits in the cupboard now and I do not feel ashamed (as many would have me feel) for not using it. There is all the food preparation and chopping to a size which will fit the fruit chute and once juice has been extracted, there are loads of movable parts of the machine which have to be washed and dried. There is a product on the market called a NutriBullet for making smoothies which my friend Kathrine Smith advocates and my proof-reader Jackie Fletcher says 'it is fab and fast and so easy to wash up!!' So if you prefer a smoothie, there is no excuse not to make one.

The goal is to put more fruit into my body and I am doing this in a way that suits me, I wash or peel the fruit and pop it into my mouth – job done!

5 **Restricted coffee and alcohol** – I love both of these and I know they are not good for my body. I gave up coffee totally during the treatment and for many years after. As you will already know I was not drinking alcohol (except champagne) until many years after the treatment had finished. 'Why go back to it?' I hear you shout. With coffee, the reason I started to drink it again was to lose weight. 'Weird' I hear you say. At the time, I was drinking over eight mugs of milky tea a day. I replaced the milky tea with black coffee and only drink it in the mornings. In the afternoon I drink unflavoured hot water. Within a few weeks, without changing anything else in my diet, I had lost half a stone in weight. For me, it is a balance between excess fat or limited diluted coffee intake.

Once I realised that my alcohol intolerance had vanished, I reintroduced some wine. I restrict my intake to one bottle per week because I do not want to overwork my liver. If there is a special occasion, then my imbibing could be more. In a normal week I will open a bottle of wine on a Friday night and when it has gone, it has gone. Sometimes it lasts until Sunday night and other times it has gone on the Friday. I really look forward to my glass of wine on a Friday night as it starts the weekend off for me. I make my decision on alcohol intake by balancing good health with good living, in my model of the world. I was born under the horoscope sign of Libra and this means I like to balance everything.

6 **Massage and love mantras** – every day when I am in the shower I perform manual lymph drainage massage on my special arm. After the massage I kiss my arm whilst at the same time saying, 'I love you.' Also during this bathroom routine, when I look in the make-up mirror I gaze directly into my eyes and tell myself, 'I love you.' This always makes me smile and is a great way to start my day.

7 **Water** – Prior to cancer I would only drink sparkling water and that was only when I was out for the evening. I was very popular because I had a lovely company car which came with free personal usage and I did not drink alcohol; so it was always my turn to drive. During a working day, I would drink between 15 to 30 machine dispensed coffees, which were delivered into a plastic cup. It never occurred to me to drink water nor did it occur to me that this drink was not coffee as it should be, it was a chemically created drink.

Nowadays it is commonly known that we should drink between 1 to 1.5 litres of water, preferably natural mineral water or filtered water, per day. This seems a lot to drink and I had to find a way to add this into my daily routine. From lunch time, I drink only hot water (except on a weekend when I imbibe some wine), or room temperature water. I fill a couple of beautiful blue glass bottles in the morning. Then I pour the water into a beautiful blue glass and I drink it throughout the day. I always drink a glass before my walk and another immediately after I return which helps with the consumption. I read somewhere (cannot remember where) that sipping water when concentrating stimulates the brain and aids concentration. I have been sipping all the time I have taken to write this book.

When I first started to drink water I thought it was very bland and I could not get used to its taste so I added lemon, orange and any other fruit I could think of to make it more palatable. Over the years I have become accustomed to the flavour of water and like it plain and simple.

8   **Pescatarian** – There are many definitions as to what this is and for me it means that I do not eat meat of any type or meat products, including chicken. I know there are those of you who realise that chicken is classified as meat but I have been asked many times, 'You do eat chicken though don't you?' and the answer is a very definite 'no.'

I do eat fish weekly, I eat dairy and eggs and loads of vegetables. I am a farmer's daughter, so being a pescatarian means I get a lot of ribbing about not eating meat, which I take on the chin. It has been suggested that dairy products are not overly good for you and being a woman of a certain age, that I should consume dairy for the calcium content, thus reducing brittle bone syndrome. As always there are contradictory viewpoints. The Libra, life in balance, comes into play, giving me choices to include dairy or not. I do keep a close eye on the amount of dairy I consume, so I manage to cover the calcium I need against the "bad fats" position. I also counter this with lots of Omega 3 oils, usually in the form of cold pressed olive oil which I love.

9   **Sugar is not always sweet** – There is now a much greater understanding of the negative role refined sugar plays in our lives and its effect on obesity, tooth decay and other related problems. The challenge is to find prepared foodstuffs without sugar. During the early years of cancer recovery I completely removed sugar from my diet. This was very hard to accomplish and I managed to do that for only two years.

Now, I give up sugar regularly and I have a much reduced sugar intake. I love chocolate and this is my nemesis. 'Get a life coach!' I hear you shout and you would be right to say this. The challenge is the pain pleasure continuum; when I am in pain I respond and when I get pleasure I respond. The effectiveness of my life coach is dependent on my position on the continuum and my sugar intake disclosure. You might find this hard to believe but I can be a little bit sneaky at times and like all drug addicts (sugar in chocolate form is my drug) hiding intake is normal, or that is my excuse.

10 **Setting daily goals** – follows on nicely from sugar intake. I always have daily goals, not in the "must be done or die" approach that some fanatical coaches adhere to but in a gently holistic approach. Some of my goals are daily ongoing as in this list and other daily goals are related to the projects I am engaged in at the time. I describe time management and goal setting in *The Business Coaching Handbook* and I use the methodologies described in my own life.

I even have goals for my weekends or holidays. They are fun goals such as planning to go on a cycle ride or to the beach. This might seem odd to those of you who are employed and therefore have weekends free. I am the owner of my own company and also an author, both of which I love to do (I get excited about my work) and because I love the job I find the lines between time off and working can sometimes get blurred. This is the reason I make goals for the weekend. I usually involve others and this commitment means I take the time off work to do different things which I enjoy. All work and no play makes Jack a dull boy and Curly a tired girl.

11 **Let it go** (this requires an open mind) – I use this technique when things are really bothering or worrying me and the same thoughts keep running around in my head. Usually negative thoughts are the ones that go round and round in my head and keep recurring. Allowing this to continue without check is one of the most energy sapping activities that happens to me. I have learnt (through continuous practise) to let go of these thoughts or worries by using a powerful technique I

learnt from a book I read by a lady called Catherine Ponder.

Now, she is a very religious person and all her books are homages to God. I do not believe in religion and I am happy to use any effective powerful technique no matter where it comes from so long as I adapt it to suit my life. Catherine Ponder's book *The Dynamic Laws of Prosperity* was recommended to me by a fellow delegate on one of the many self and wealth development courses I attended. When I first started to read the book I had to use all my powers of self-control to enable me to get past the God stuff. I learnt to replace the word God with universe and this made life a lot easier. Ponder has many very useful sayings and incantations – I have adapted one of my favourites using the word universe as a substitute for the word God:

'I loosen and let go. I let go and let the universe's love do its perfect work in me, through me, for me. I let go and let the universe's love do its perfect work in the conscious, subconscious and super conscious activities of my mind, body and affairs. I give thanks that peace, health, plenty and happiness now reign supreme in me and in my world.'

I realise this is a bit long and takes some learning and practice for it to trip off the tongue easily. At first, I just used to say the starting sentence, 'I loosen and let go,' over and over again. I blocked the other thoughts from coming into my mind. I would keep doing this in my head or aloud, until the other thoughts lost their hold on my mind. It is a really freeing experience being in control and able to release negative thoughts and worries.

Here is another of Catherine Ponder's sayings which I have also adapted:

'(Name of person) I fully and freely forgive you. I loosen you, and let you go. So far as I am concerned, that incident between us is finished forever. I do not wish to hurt you. I wish you no harm. I am free and you are free and all is again well between us.'

I find this saying very powerful when I feel an injustice has been done to me, where I continually run conversations I had with the person, or conversations I am planning to have with this person, in my mind. Often, after saying this a few times the person calls and rectifies the problem. A mini miracle. Either way, I always end up feeling better about myself and the situation.

12 **Skin Creams** – the skin is the largest organ in our bodies, which is pretty obvious when you think about it. During my treatment for cancer at the Royal Marsden Hospital, a nurse asked me, 'Do you use body cream as a daily routine?' and I said not really and I followed this with the question, 'Why?'

She said, 'Your skin needs nourishment especially during the cancer treatments and I strongly recommend you start using a body cream.' She also mentioned that the body is doing a lot of healing at this time and if you put cream on your skin, it is one thing less for the body to have to deal with. How simple and effective is that? I now use cream (not Devon Clotted Cream as used on scones in a cream tea) or body milk on my skin every day so that my body can be healing other areas which I might not know about. I prefer chemical free body oils or lotions as there are some real nasties in everyday body products. Currently there are few or no restrictions about what can go into an external body product. Just think about that sentence. It is quite daunting and scary when you realise the lack of regulation and the opportunity for exploitation in this area.

Apparently, there is this stuff called Sodium Lauryl Sulphate or SLS for short. It has been known to cause irritation of the skin, eyes, and also in some cases, lungs. When mixed with other chemicals (I do not know which chemicals nor if these chemicals are commonly found in or around the human body – therefore I do not know the level of risk) can form nitrosamines and most of these are carcinogenic. I was amazed at how many of the products in my bathroom cabinet contained SLS.

The above list of daily dozen is really my blueprint lifestyle plan and it is now part and parcel of who I am and what I do. The above dozen happen naturally, I do not have to think about them because I have made them into natural habits, things that happen without my needing to concentrate on them.

SUMMING UP

As this chapter is all about summing up activities I have decided not to create a summing up list. I have taken the time to create a daily dozen as a maintenance plan for consistent good health and I have integrated this plan into my life. It is easy to do and easy to remember.

Epilogue

LOOSE ENDS

What happened since?

I was going to end the book on chapter 20, *The daily dozen*, as it seemed to me to be a brief summary of all that is in the book. However my early readers asked me questions which started with 'What happened to …?' so I felt I needed to tie up some of the loose ends.

'What happened to Faisal?' one of the early readers asked. For those of you who have forgotten who Faisal was, he was the doctor friend who let me stay at his house and who managed to get me an appointment with the Royal Marsden Hospital. He was also my bridesmaid when Pete and I married. Well he is now a senior partner of the Bush Doctors in Shepherds Bush and is happily married to an old sweetheart from his medical school days.

'What happened to your mother?' My mother is still alive and imbibing whiskey. It is her 90th birthday this year and by the time the book has gone to publication we will have had the party to celebrate her achievement. Already 70 people have RSVP'd saying they are coming and that tells you all you need to know about her popularity. She is the most amazing person I know and I have dedicated books to her. I know I am lucky on many levels; she is still alive, she dresses elegantly, she still puts on make-up, she still drives safely, she still has all her faculties, she still does crosswords, she is the "go-to" person for troubled souls and she makes us all laugh. How lucky am I to have been born to her?

'What happened to your hair?' I have often been asked about my hair since the chemotherapy and to summarise, I kept it short for many years (about 16 years or so) as I was used to short spiky hair and it was very easy to manage. I had lost the thickness and the strength of the hair so I decided to keep it short in the hope it would remain healthy. Interestingly, I would still have short hair if two things had not happened within close timing of each other. The first was a picture taken of me, side on when I was delivering a public speech about the benefits of life coaching; I noticed that my hair looked ridiculous. I was nearing my sixties and still had spikey short hair and I did not like the overall impression.

Then shortly after, I was involved in a very serious cycling accident, so serious I was airlifted to the nearest accident and emergency department in a coma. I had been cycling down a country lane travelling at about 20-25 miles per hour and skidded on gravel whilst manoeuvring around a sharp right hand bend. I cannot remember anything about the accident, I shattered my right shoulder and I travelled along the tarmac on my face! The trauma was so bad I could not wash my hair for quite some time and I decided that I would let it grow. I now have shoulder length hair and I love it. It is still a bit thin on the crown and this is covered by a fringe. Every cloud has a silver lining.

Since the massage I had at the Royal Marsden Hospital I have always had regular massages because of the huge benefits to my body. I have often volunteered to be the model for massage students as I remember how hard it was to qualify when I did the course. My current masseuse was a student when we first met and I was a volunteer for her. She is now qualified and studying for a sports massage qualification. There is always something for her to work on as I have usually done something to my body between visits and she can practise her new sports massage techniques. The thing is that it is most unlikely that I would ever have had a massage if I had not been given the opportunity from the Royal Marsden Hospital, which also means that cancer was the catalyst for this joyful and healthy form of therapy.

Talking of therapies I have been asked, 'What therapies have you continued or experienced since the cancer?' As I mention above, I continue to have regular massage. I continue to use laughter therapy in a daily integrated way and by selecting to watch comedy movies and read books which have been reviewed as "side-splitting" as this always helps to keep the body healed. Also, I have heard about some recent research which claims that cuddling is good for you – so I do a lot of that! Usually I only cuddle the people that I already know.

The beautiful side effect of being diagnosed with cancer for me was the opening of my mind. This has led me to investigate, explore and experience a wide variety of things which, without the cancer, I would most probably not have experienced because, as I have previously mentioned, I was very narrow minded and bigoted. What is important for me is that I tried lots of different things, at differing times, during the 20 year period. This means I am unable to state categorically that one therapy worked and another did not. Here are the therapies I tried.

Feng Shui is an ancient Chinese custom of organising your home and your work environment to foster health, happiness, and wealth. I looked into this and decided to rearrange my furniture according to the directions. I think it works, only it is hard to judge or measure as the feelings are subjective because Feng Shui promotes a healthy flow of chi and it increases the vital energy within the building. I do however take into consideration the Feng Shui directions every time I move house, so I suppose I am a believer or is it because I like to stack the odds in my favour. Who knows?

I was taught Hypnotherapy as part of the NLP master practitioner course I attended. This therapy uses speech as a way to bypass the conscious mind and access the inner or subconscious mind. It can facilitate changes such as weight loss, anxiety, phobias or smoking cessation. I have used hypnosis with my coaching clients (with their permission) to great effect.

I also learnt how to perform Reflexology on another course. This therapy uses the fingers and thumbs of the practitioner who applies pressure to points on the feet or hands to treat a wide range of illnesses. This therapy is based on the premise that specific points on the feet and hands correspond with organs and tissues in the body. When pressure is applied to the points on the feet or hands, if the therapist feels a grit-like nodule in any spot they know which part of the body is not functioning properly. The idea is that the therapist can massage away the grit and this can heal the body part. It seemed to work for me; I could definitely feel the grit when I performed the reflexology. I did this for a short while as I was not considering this as a career move – I was just curious.

I have tried the Bach Flower Remedies which are mostly aimed at curing emotional states rather than physical ones. I cannot claim that they have worked magic for me, just that I have tried them. The lack of proof of efficacy might be due to the fact that I constantly guard my thoughts and use visualisation and affirmations on a daily basis, so I am able to control my emotional states anyway.

I have consulted with a Chiropractor, although I did find the treatment was a bit rough and it pulled me about a bit more than I was comfortable with. This might be due to the scars from the operation making lying on my front unpleasant. I have had a much more effective result from Spinal Touch Therapy, which is a gentle yet powerful treatment for backache and muscular skeletal complaints. It is all about the gravitational pull on the skeleton and the way the therapist rebalances the effects of the gravitational pull.

One of the fast change therapies I love is called Emotional Freedom Techniques or EFT for short. Some of you might know it as the tapping therapy because it involves gently tapping specific areas around the body. I was introduced to this therapy by a very dear friend Ric Hayman who has a brain the size of a planet and a heart to match. Not only is he a genius with computers he is also one of the most curious people I know. He will dig around, poke into, search out and pursue anything that might be useful to his family, his friends, his coaching clients and himself. If you have not experienced EFT then I recommend you look into it.

I did have Shiatsu during my recovery. I cannot say if it had any effect on my healing process although it did work on my easing my back ache. Shiatsu is a type of acupressure which has been performed in Japan for over 1,000 years. It is used to ease pain, stimulate the body's natural energies and for general health maintenance. What made the sessions more interesting is that the practitioner was a druid and he attended the solstice celebrations at Stonehenge. We had many a thought provoking chat pre and post Shiatsu session.

There is a term called Vitamin Therapy which quite surprised me as I had been taking vitamins and minerals almost from the start of the cancer diagnosis. I stumbled on this title which seems to describe the use of vitamins in a combined form to enhance the body's ability to combat diseases. I do this as you already know from my chapters and from the daily dozen chapter.

'What happened to facial tanning?' I still use facial quick tan as a boost and I also put my make-up on to go to town or out of the locality. I immediately feel enhanced and elevated in mood and well-being. This could of course be the result of my anticipation in leaving the home to go out for a while, although I strongly expect it is the combination of the expectation of going out and the application of make-up together providing the catalyst for euphoria. I am easily happy. I still look like a carrot on the occasions where I am a little more enthusiastic with the tanning cream and that is okay with me and gives my friends and family something to smile about.

'What has happened to all the people who attended the farewell party?' Well some of them are sadly no longer with us. Some have moved away out of my sphere and the rest are still in contact and attending the mad family and friend parties we hold.

I continue to keep my teeth mercury free and I have to say I am impressed with the longevity of the composite fillings. I have never regretted the removal of the mercury ones.

I dedicated an entire chapter to the menopause and for the most part I still suffer from the power surges (hot flushes) day and night and most of the other symptoms which come with menopause. I have learnt to accept them as part of my life as I have tried many of the therapies and remedies which are within my oestrogen positive restricted list to little or no avail. After so long it is probably safe for me to have the oestrogen creams or HRT, only life is great as it is, so when I ask myself 'Why take the risk?' the answer is always 'There are no reasons to take a risk with health.'

Last but not least I need to write a bit about Pete. He started as my boyfriend who could not handle the fact that I had been diagnosed with cancer. We parted company at Malaga airport and he followed me to the UK and asked to be forgiven and taken back, which I agreed to. It is interesting that looking back on the events with hindsight to the cancer announcement, I discovered many people cannot deal with it or they react to the information in unusual ways.

Whilst I was having the chemotherapy Pete was training to become an electrician. He noticed that in my bedroom I only had one socket from which I had extension leads to the many electrical appliances a lady needs. One weekend, he propelled me out of my sick bed into the front room where he had opened the sofa bed and arranged the bedding for me to move into. He did this with the true sergeant major efficiency he was used to employing with his company of marines.

Then with the gusto I would later become accustomed to, he proceeded to empty my bedroom by putting everything in the hallway and all around me in my front room. Then he took up the carpet and removed the floor boards!

My flat was heated by electric storage heaters and because Pete needed to turn the electric off for safety reasons it rapidly became very cold. Picture this for a moment; I am lying in bed wearing a winter coat, a knitted bobble hat, a scarf and a pair of gloves under the duvet. When I mentioned to Pete that there was perhaps a better time to add sockets to my bedroom he was amazed and could not understand how I was nowhere near as enthusiastic as he was, as I so clearly needed extra sockets. After two days in the front room and the addition of eight double sockets to my bedroom it was all over. I even had sockets in the wardrobe!

After all the chemotherapy and radiotherapy had finished I was about to start looking for a job and Pete and I had a discussion about my moving to Bournemouth where he was based. I started to look for apartments to rent in the Bournemouth area (I was not ready to commit to fully moving to Bournemouth). I have no idea how it happened but I ended up buying a house with him. Whilst showing potential buyers around my flat in London, when we reached the bedroom, the same question was asked each time, "Why have you got so many sockets?" I would answer, "My boyfriend is an electrician."

After I had moved into the house I found work as a freelance trainer and settled down living with Pete; he proposed seven years later and we were married much to the amazement of all our friends. We are still together and live in the West Country. The moral of this little story is that if you can forgive, (you might have to forgive many things) sometimes the rewards of forgiving are ongoing. This of course also includes forgiving your body for the disease and forgiving yourself for everything.

Just a last thought, which I was reminded of by a friend and I had completely forgotten about, is an affirmation or incantation which I used at the time. I would say often throughout the day, 'Thank you dear cancer, your service to me is now complete, I release you and set you free and myself free. We are both free and it is done.'

Thank you for spending time with me and I wish you health, wealth and abundant happiness.

About The Author

Curly Martin was diagnosed with breast cancer, and an aggressive form of lymphatic cancer 1992 and she was given nine months to live. At that time she became homeless and was unemployed. Since then she has become the international bestselling author of, *The Coaching Handbook Series* of books. *The Life Coaching Handbook* was a world first, a book written for coaches about the business of coaching. *The Business Coaching Handbook* came next, followed by *The Personal Success Handbook*; all her books are greatly acclaimed.

She is a highly sought-after international speaker, a pioneer of life coaching in Europe and the founder of a very successful coach training company, Achievement Specialists Limited. She intuitively combines her personal experiences with accepted methodologies and cutting edge innovations, to create exciting, entertaining and effective approaches to personal success and development.

In her books, she shares all the knowledge, tips and secrets that she discovered during her life journey, including techniques and strategies she used to overcome her physical challenges and how she now lives a passionate, exciting, wealthy, healthy, happy and spiritual life. Curly would love to hear from you.

How To Contact Curly

When you are ready and want to discover more about my journey, or to receive support through coaching, please visit my webpages: *www.curlymartin.com*

How To Become A Life Coach

If you are interested in becoming a life coach or cancer coach visit: *www.achievementspecialists.co.uk.*

Achievement Specialists offers one of the most advanced Life Coaching training courses available, based on the ground-breaking work in this area The Life Coaching Handbook. Everything you need to be an effective Life Coach. Author Curly Martin. The course we offer has been accredited level 7 by the International Institute of Coaching & Mentoring, it is a fully integrated, blended, multi-media, supported and flexible diploma. Curly delivers the course so you are trained by her.

Acknowledgements

Thank you to all of the people I have mentioned within this book.

Thank you to my pre-release readers. Your comments and Moji's made me laugh. Your attention to detail and your generosity astounded me. I thank you all from the bottom (not quite sure about the use of the word bottom) of my heart.

Shirley Aubrey, Ann Beatty, Jackie Fletcher, Pete Frizzel, Cathy Fulgar, Prue Gent, Sue Greenaway, Georg Guy, Jackie Hammans, Jenny Heath, Tolga Kulahcigil, Professor Angus McLeod, Elizabeth Rankich, Kathrine Smith, Chris Striblehill, Antonia Swinton, Grant Willcox.

Thank you to Salli Griffith for the cover design, she is wonderful to work with.

Thank you to Ric Hayman for his friendship, for putting together the new website in time for the book launch *www.curlymartin.com* and his valuable support in all things technical.

Thank you to Keith Down for giving me a place to write and for taking the cover photograph.

Thank you to Phil and Jo Down for the loan of a camera.

Thank you Ray Brooks for your hospitality in keeping me fed during the mammoth writing month.

Thank you to Pete for steering and steadying the ship.

Testimonials For Curly Martin

'Curly, your skills, knowledge and wisdom have changed and transformed my world. I thank you for all your guidance this past year and your love for making a difference to so many lives. You are a star!'

—K. COTTAM

'No words could express my gratitude firstly, for your book that opened the door for me and so many others and for your gift of magic that you have poured on us all. To live in this new place is indescribable. It carries with it a sense of dignity and ease that I have never ever envisaged. From my heart I thank God for it and I thank you also Curly.'

—MARY BURKE

'Dear Curly, It was a real pleasure to meet you. As I mentioned, your energy is amazing and you really inspire. I thoroughly enjoyed the course, in fact the best personal development course I've been on. I learnt a lot about myself even though I was doing things outside my comfort zone, I felt real warmth, support and encouragement from everyone and the feedback was always very constructive and helpful, in terms of improving in the future. Thanks again for a fun and very inspiring weekend!'

—JOANNA PUCZKOWSKI

'I just wanted to say thank you so much – it was truly a life changing experience. I burst into tears of utter joy this morning as I was dancing my bum off around the kitchen to Heather Small singing 'Proud'. Being a verbose individual, I could go on and on about it all but I'm not going to. What I'm going to do is get my 'arris into gear and get on with it! Thank you again, Curly.'

—M. PHELPS

'A supremely powerful learning experience – more than exceeded my expectations. Jam-packed with useful information and practical advice. I highly recommend this opportunity to anyone wanting to enhance their own personal life and business and management skills. You will thoroughly enjoy, and benefit from this unique experience. I am positive that you will come out of this two-day event with the belief that absolutely anything you chose, and dare to dream, is within your grasp.'

—TANYA PALMER

'It has now been over 2 weeks since I participated on your brilliant Life course. Thank you so much for a great course, practical and thought provoking. And wow! I have achieved loads in the last 2 weeks. I am so focussed and results driven – and this is in all aspects of my life, we are eating better; I am keeping fit, I have completed tasks that I have been procrastinating for weeks; (including my tax return); and I feel good (in a James Brown style!) Thank you Curly – you are an inspiration. Warmest Regards'

—LINDSEY REED

'LOVED EVERYTHING! Thank you Curly, you are truly an inspiration. This has given me the confidence to be the best person that I can be.'

—CAROLE GERRO

'Just wanted to say thank you. I was very impressed. As you know I taught in colleges for 8 years and have been to many talks conferences trainings etc., yours would have to be No 1 because I learnt so much. You kept my attention. Timings were excellent and you delivered what you said you would. Thanks.'

—GENEEN CROSSLEY

عزيـزتي كـــيرلي،

أكتـب لك هذها الرسـالة. لـعبر عن مدى شكري وامتنـانـي لمسـا ا لعدلة
تـي قـدمتها لـي أثنـاء إ تبـاعي دورةا لـدوم في بلـرل التطويـر ا ذاتي.

عندما قـررت الانضمامإلى الـدورة كنـت فيـأ سـواً حـالاتلي نا سـفية
فقـد كنـت تعرضـت لخسـارة كبـي رقفيـا لعمـل علـا وملسـتوى
الاجتماعي مماأ شـعرنيب الهزيمـاة لـوفش لـبي بـا فقـدانل ثقـة ا
ا بلـذاتو القـدرة علـا ل امتبعـة. و هأانا الآن بعـد

طبريقـةإ الأمور برؤيـة وقد شـره عشـرةأ حصـلت علـا لبـدلوم نـوا قلبـت يـا حتي أ رسـا على
عقـب. ف قـدا دسـتتع تقتيـل بنـافس وبـدأت برؤيـة
يجـا أكـثر بيـة ف لكـل وضـع هناكا لكثـير سـلبل منـا علاجل المشـاكل
وأكـثر رطيقـة لمـوا جهةل تحـديات ا.

لاقسـد تمتعـت بكـل قرأتـه تكـاب أثنـاءا الـدرا سة سـوتفدت من كل ا
الخطوات ا ولم ه امت الظويفيـة الـتي تـوج بعلينـا أداؤ ها أ ثنـاء ا تـا
بعـ الـدورة.

عإجابيـب الـدورة وم بفهومـا لتطويـرا لـذا ديفعانيا تـ للـى تـافكير
جـديا بطـرح الـدورب ةاالعربيـة للغـة لعربيـة نشـر هذاا ملفهومـا د ل جيـد لاقـديم
ا ولـذي مازال جديـدا وغـير مطرو قفيـا الـدانا بللـ لعربيـة.

أ تمـنى لكـك ل تويفـق ولن أ تـرد دعلى الإطلاقـت بقـديم النصـيحة
لأي ا شخص هـذ تبـاعا الدورلة تحقيـق مسـتقبل أ فضـل أ

Other Books by Curly Martin

The Life Coaching Handbook. Everything You
Need To Be An Effective Life Coach.

The Business Coaching Handbook. Everything
You Need To Be Your Own Business Coach.

The Personal Success Handbook. Everything
You Need To Be Successful.

Readers Bonus Gift

As an extra thank you for purchasing this book I offer you a bonus gift from my Health Download To Destiny (D2D) E-series of programmes.

Visit *www.curlymartin.com/bonus* to claim your gift.

Lightning Source UK Ltd.
Milton Keynes UK
UKOW05f1900130217

294320UK00020B/713/P